5548

Withdrawn

Handbook for the
Hospital Medical Secretary

Handbook for the Hospital Medical Secretary

JOAN GRIFFITHS

MEDICAL ADVISOR:
BOYD S GOLDIE

BSc, FRCS, DHMSA
Orthopaedic Senior Registrar
Royal London Hospital

OXFORD
BLACKWELL SCIENTIFIC PUBLICATIONS
LONDON EDINBURGH BOSTON
MELBOURNE PARIS BERLIN VIENNA

Blackwell Scientific Publications
Editorial Offices:
Osney Mead, Oxford OX2 0EL
25 John Street, London WC1N 2BL
23 Ainslie Place, Edinburgh EH3 6AJ
238 Main Street, Cambridge
  Massachusetts 02142, USA
54 University Street, Carlton
  Victoria 3053, Australia

Other Editorial Offices:
Librairie Arnette SA
2, rue Casimir-Delavigne
75006 Paris
France

Blackwell Wissenschafts-Verlag GmbH
Meinekestrasse 4
D-1000 Berlin 15
Germany

Blackwell MZV
Feldgasse 13
A-1238 Wien
Austria

First published 1993

Set by Best-set Typesetter Ltd., Hong
Kong
Printed and bound in Great Britain by
Hartnolls Ltd, Bodmin, Cornwall

DISTRIBUTORS

Marston Book Services Ltd
PO Box 87
Oxford OX2 0DT
(Orders: Tel: 0865 791155
        Fax: 0865 791927
        Telex: 837515)

USA
Blackwell Scientific Publications, Inc.
238 Main Street
Cambridge, MA 02142
(Orders: Tel: 800 759-6102
             617 876-7000)

Canada
Times Mirror Professional Publishing, Ltd
130 Flaska Drive
Markham, Ontario L6G 1B8
(Orders: Tel: 800 268-4178
             416 470-6739)

Australia
Blackwell Scientific Publications Pty Ltd
54 University Street
Carlton, Victoria 3053
(Orders: Tel: 03 347-5552)

British Library
Cataloguing in Publication Data

A catalogue record for this title
is available from the British Library

0-632-03584-6

Library of Congress
Cataloging in Publication Data

Griffiths, Joan.
    Handbook for the hospital medical
secretary/Joan Griffiths.
        p.   cm.
    Includes bibliographical references
and index.
    ISBN 0-632-03584-6
    1. Hospital secretaries – Handbooks,
manuals, etc.   2. Medical secretaries –
Handbooks, manuals, etc.
3. Medicine – Terminology.   I. Title.
    [DNLM: 1. Medical Secretaries –
handbooks.   W 39 G855h 1993]
RA972.55.G74   1993
651.9′36211 – dc20   93-12007   CIP

Contents

Preface

The medical secretary working in hospital will find this book of great value. It is the first to have been written exclusively for the hospital medical secretary. It will be particularly useful to the temporary secretary who is called upon to work in any speciality at short notice. In addition, it is a useful resource for those undertaking a formal training.

The contents embrace a wide field. Departments and staff within the hospital setting are introduced; basic anatomical terms are explained and the importance of mastering medical terminology emphasized. The main specialities are covered in detail and are richly illustrated with samples of letters and reports.

The book's value for reference purposes is amply shown in the chapter relating to investigations and in the list of medical diagnoses, abbreviations, surgical operations and terms applicable to each speciality. Much of this information will also be of help to hospital clerical workers especially medical records staff.

For ease of reference the book is divided into four parts:

Part I   The Secretary and the Hospital – This covers the secretary's duties, the various departments and staff within the hospital, including administrative, medical, nursing, allied professions and support staff.

Part II   Medical Basics – This explains the various systems of the body, introducing root words, prefixes and suffixes, and covering medical investigations and drugs.

Part III   Terminology for General Medicine and Surgery – This provides the essential terms with which every medical secretary should be familiar, with many samples of medical and surgical summaries and X-ray reports.

Part IV   Terminology for Specialities – This incorporates the terminology of the main specialities, with lists of terms and abundant samples of letters and reports. In the surgical specialities, lists of operations are included. This information will be invaluable to the relief secretary and a vital source of reference to all secretaries.

At the back of the book there is a further selection of medical terms listed alphabetically with word elements for quick reference.

Joan Griffiths

Part I
The Secretary and the Hospital

Chapter 1
The Secretary in Different Departments

Secretarial posts in large general hospitals vary widely. Many require a good working knowledge of medical terminology and procedure; others are more suitable for novices. Some secretaries meet with the patient or have considerable telephone contact, whereas others may have no personal involvement at all. However, most posts are busy, and carry a high level of responsibility.

Before applying for a medical secretarial post it is important to find out as much as possible about the particular job. Also, ask yourself whether it is a job that holds real interest and appeal for you, and whether it lies within your capability. To be of real value, the secretary should also know the terminology and procedures of the department to which they are being sent.

This chapter briefly outlines the various hospital departments and specialities and looks at the role of the secretary within these. Specific duties are dealt with in Chapter 2. First, however, it is necessary to look at the two broad categories of hospital specialities, medical and surgical. Most departments came under one or other 'field', although there is obviously an area of overlap in many instances.

The medical field

This encompasses the non-surgical treatment of disease and comprises those specialities where treatment is usually by drugs (rather than surgery) and the condition frequently (but by no means always) **chronic** – i.e. long-standing and on-going – for example, rheumatology.

Medicine attracts 'general' as well as 'specialist' physicians.

chronic (a term applied to a disease or disorder) developing slowly and persisting for a long time. Opposite of **acute**.

medicine in this context, the practice of treating illness and disease without surgery. (Also a remedy for illness.)

General physicians

The general physician as the name implies, covers the general medical treatment of all systems of the body but they may have special interest and

3

experience in for example chest conditions, heart, hypertension (high blood pressure), endocrinology, urology or gastroenterology. There are normally about three or four general physicians in a district general hospital. Some knowledge of drugs is particularly useful in general medicine. As well as general medical terminology the secretary needs to be familiar with types of investigations and some common operative procedures, for example, endoscopy.

The surgical field

Here the treatment of disease is by surgical methods and tends to include more 'acute' i.e. urgent and immediate cases.

acute   (a term applied to a disease or its symptoms) beginning suddenly and with marked intensity. Although it lasts for a short period of time it often requires emergency treatment.
surgery   the branch of medicine treating disease by operative techniques (adjective = surgical).

General surgeons

The general surgeon performs general surgical procedures such as hernia repairs, removal of gall bladder, appendix, stomach and bowel, but they also have their own special interest and skills, perhaps for breast, gastric, urological or vascular surgery. Many patients under the care of the general surgeon have malignant tumours removed and therefore require regular follow up. Minor surgical procedures may be carried out on a day-care basis with the patient arriving and leaving on the same day. Many hospitals have a Surgical Day Unit especially for this purpose with its own nursing, clerical and possibly secretarial staff.

Neurosurgery (brain and nerve surgery), cardiac surgery, kidney and other transplant surgery are normally carried out in specialist units and the secretary attached to these needs to be experienced in medical secretarial duties and familiar with specialist terminology.

Hospital departments and specialities

Accident and Emergency (A & E or Casualty)

This department is at the forefront of hospital care – though these days located only in large hospitals. This is where people who have had serious accidents or who are suddenly and/or severely ill are brought for medical attention – either by ambulance or by themselves. It is perhaps the busiest department, open 24 hours, 365 days a year.

The consultant doctor in charge of this department may be either a physician or a surgeon as emergencies coming through Accident and Emergency/Casualty may be of a medical or surgical nature. Any patient subsequently admitted to the hospital comes under the care of the appropriate consultant according to the nature of the patient's condition. The Accident and Emergency consultant does not usually have beds in the hospital.

Because of the acute nature of this department, there is usually only a part-time secretary; formal secretarial duties are hardly required. Letters of notification to the GPs of patients attending are usually written, speedily, by hand by the junior medical staff. In some hospitals word processors are used by the nursing and medical staff to up-date records and write letters. Most correspondence is about accident cases not admitted, insurance claims, and referral letters to other consultants' outpatient clinics.

Anaesthetics

Anaesthetics is the branch of medicine concerned with the relief of pain and the administration of pain-relieving drugs and life-support measures during surgery. In a district general hospital there would probably be at least six consultant anaesthetists supported by a team of more junior doctors. Usually the department office is situated next to the operating theatres where the anaesthetists' work is centred. The secretary to the Anaesthetic Department is often a part-time post. Medical terminology, although useful, is not necessary as the secretary's task mainly consists of organizing the doctors' on-call rotas, making arrangements for a temporary ('locum') anaesthetist to cover someone away on holiday or off sick, dealing with travel and other expenses claims, general correspondence, occasional medical reports, and perhaps the minutes of meetings. In some hospitals, the anaesthetic secretary types out the list of patients' names and record numbers (known as 'The List') for the next day's operations. It is very important that there are no errors in this list. Sometimes a consultant anaesthetist may, in addition to working in theatre, run a pain clinic (for people suffering from intractable pain) or attend a clinic where surgeons refer their 'at risk' patients (e.g. those with long-standing chest complaints) to be assessed for suitability of receiving an anaesthetic. As these are likely to be the only outpatient clinics attached to the department, the anaesthetic secretary will have no direct patient contact.

In some hospitals the consultant in charge of the Intensive Care (or Therapy) Unit (ICU or ITU) is an anaesthetist as many patients will be on breathing machines (ventilators) and heavily sedated.

Cardiology

This is the heart speciality. Patients suffering from cardiovascular diseases (diseases of the heart and its vessels) are referred by their GP to the cardiology clinic where they are seen by the heart specialist (cardiologist). In some hospitals general physicians look after patients with cardiovascular problems but in many large hospitals there is a specialist physician who deals with cardiac cases only.

Cardiology is a high-powered speciality involving both medical and surgical treatments. A good knowledge of cardiac terminology – and abbreviations – is important.

Dermatology

Dermatology refers to the skin, and a specialist physician (dermatologist) treats diseases of the skin. As most patients are treated on an outpatient basis, the number of beds allocated to the dermatologist in a general hospital are usually quite few. If surgery is required for **biopsy** or removal of **lesions**, the patient may be referred to the plastic or general surgeon. The terminology is quite specialized as there are many dermatological diseases and terms to describe the appearance of the skin (see Chapter 13).

biopsy   removal of a small sample of living tissue for diagnosis.
lesion   any wound, injury or abnormal change to body tissue.

Ear, Nose and Throat (ENT)

The secretary who works in this department should have some knowledge of the anatomy of the ear, nose, throat, sinuses and ENT operations. Quite a large proportion of the patients are children, requiring grommet tube insertion for fluid in the middle ear, sinus washouts or the removal of tonsils and adenoids.

However, adult patients of every age can suffer a variety of ENT problems such as nasal polyps, ear and sinus infections, vocal nodules and tumours.

Endocrinology

This department is concerned with the endocrine (hormonal) system (see Chapter 5) and the treatment of patients with problems or diseases in this system. An example of two very common conditions are diabetes and thyroid disorders. The endocrinologist usually treats a wide range of general medical problems as well so the secretary must be familiar with general medicine terminology.

Gastroenterology

This busy department will be involved in the care of those with ailments affecting any part of their alimentary/gastrointestinal tract. Thus, patients will include those with stomach and duodenal ulcers, gallstones, diarrhoea and constipation, irritable bowel syndrome as well as food sensitivities and allergies like coeliac disease.

Genetics

Some hospitals have a consultant geneticist or there may be a visiting one. This specialty is the study of genes and inherited diseases. The department will offer counselling services (for example, preconceptual counselling in cases of a family history of inherited disease) as well as diagnostic and screening measures.

Genitourinary Medicine

This department is concerned with genital diseases (sexually transmitted diseases), bladder and urinary problems in both sexes, and prostate and reproductive troubles in males. Thus, it combines the previously separate Sexually Transmitted Diseases and Urology departments.

The consultant physician who heads this department is likely to be a specialist in sexually transmitted diseases – and this would include AIDS. In this instance, it is usually possible for patients to attend the clinics held without GP referral.

Gynaecology and Obstetrics

Gynaecology is the study of woman's reproductive organs and their diseases (and overlap, with endocrinology in this respect); obstetrics is concerned with the medical and surgical management of pregnancy and parturition (delivery).

There would probably be three consultant gynaecologists/obstetricians in a district general hospital with about 450 beds and, depending on the size of the obstetric unit; there may be a secretary wholly for obstetrics. However, if the maternity unit is quite small, with not more than 1500 deliveries a year, the secretarial work is normally undertaken by the secretary working for her individual consultant in his gynaecological capacity. Much of this work is so closely interlinked that in many cases this is a more satisfactory arrangement. For example, patients are usually admitted to the gynaecological wards who miscarry, or threaten to miscarry, or develop some early complication of pregnancy; they are only admitted to the maternity wards at a later stage when the fetus is viable. Terminations of pregnancy (TOPs) are also carried out in the gynaecology department.

The gynaecological unit is a very busy one with a high turnover of patients, as many are admitted for minor surgical procedures and discharged the following day. There are usually a large number of telephone calls regarding operation dates, admissions, appointments, results of tests and from Medical Records looking for notes. If medical students are attached to the Obstetric Unit, the secretary may be required to do some administrative duties regarding their rotas etc.

Typing minutes of meetings and preparing reports for the monthly Perinatal Mortality Meeting, which is held in most Obstetric Units, will almost certainly be some of the other tasks.

Neurology

Neurology is to do with the brain, the spinal cord and the rest of the nervous system. The neurologist will be concerned with diseases of the central nervous system, such as multiple sclerosis and Parkinson's disease, and anything which affects the proper functioning of the body's nerves – whether the result of tumours, trauma, or ageing.

Again the secretary needs to know general medicine terminology as the doctors on the team are sometimes on call for the general medical wards.

Ophthalmology

This is the eye speciality. Although there are eye departments within many general hospitals, some districts have a completely separate eye hospital with its own beds, theatres, Outpatient, Accident and Emergency, X-ray and Medical Records departments, and all the necessary staff to manage a self-contained acute hospital. Those referred for the suitability of being granted a driving licence are tested here, and there is special equipment for testing for night- and colour-blindness. Thus, dark rooms with television screens, lasers and microscopes feature largely in an ophthalmic unit.

As well as the consultant ophthalmologist and the junior medical team, there will be an orthoptist – an expert in the technique of eye exercises to correct the visual axes of eyes not properly co-ordinated (orthoptics). Many of the orthoptist's patients are children with varying degrees of strabismus (squint). There may also be an optician, with perhaps a small shop and a display of frames, or an optometrist – a technician trained in optics and certain phases of refraction.

The secretary working for the ophthalmologist and the junior medical team should be familiar with the basic anatomical terms referring to the eye as well as the words used to describe the various signs, symptoms and diseases of the eye.

Oral surgery

Large district general hospitals usually have an Oral Maxillofacial Surgery unit. Some teaching hospitals have a dental school attached, and it is usually only in these hospitals that emergency dental treatment can be obtained through the Accident and Emergency department.

In an Oral Maxillofacial department there would be a number of consultant oral surgeons. Much of their work is involved in difficult extraction of teeth, such as impacted wisdom teeth (eights), jaw surgery for abnormalities or following fractures, removal of tumours and dealing with injuries and infection in the maxillofacial region. They have their own team of junior doctors.

Also attached to the Oral Surgery department would be specialists in orthodontics, that is the branch of dentistry which deals with the development, prevention and correction of irregularities of the teeth and mal-occlusion. Most of the patients are children and the orthodontist, in cases of overcrowding of teeth, will advise the child's dental surgeon which teeth to extract and what appliance to use to correct the malocclusion.

The department would also have specialist dental surgeons in restorative dentistry and highly qualified dental technicians and possibly a senior chief maxillofacial technologist. In addition to the medical/dental staff there would be dental nurses, hygienists, secretaries and receptionists.

It is helpful for the secretary to be familiar with the anatomical terms relating to the face and jaw and to know some dental terminology.

Orthopaedics

Orthopaedic surgery is the surgery of the musculoskeletal system – i.e. bones, joints, muscles and nerves. There is overlap between orthopaedic surgery and plastic surgery in the care of conditions of the hand and there is overlap with neurology and the neurosurgeons in the care of spine and spinal cord. Orthopaedic surgery includes 'cold' surgery (also known as 'elective') such as total hip replacement, and trauma which mainly comprises fractures which may or may not require inpatient care.

The secretary who works in the orthopaedic department should be familiar with the anatomical terms of the musculoskeletal system and much of the terminology relevant to rheumatology is useful to the orthopaedic secretary. There is close liaison between the physical medicine/rheumatology consultant and the orthopaedic surgeon, and sometimes they hold combined clinics.

As patients with fractures form a large group of those under the care of the Orthopaedic department, special fracture clinics are held – perhaps twice or three times a week, or even daily. Those who come to Accident and Emergency with fractures but not needing admission are usually given an appointment for the next fracture clinic so that the diagnosis and treatment of the fracture can be checked (it will have been dealt with in Accident and Emergency/Casualty); thereafter patients are looked after by the orthopaedic team. The plaster technician and physiotherapists are also very much involved in the care of patients with fractures.

In most units clinic notes, operation notes and the results of consultant ward rounds are dictated and then typed into the patient's notes. In a few units, even the doctor's inpatient notes are typed out. Consequently, orthopaedic secretaries often have a large amount of copy-typing to do. Some consultants like their secretaries to sit in with them in the outpatient clinic and accompany them on the ward rounds and take shorthand. When in clinic, there may be considerable interaction with patients, which many secretaries enjoy.

Some orthopaedic patients may benefit from the orthotic service (surgical appliances), especially in cases of back injuries when surgical corsets may be prescribed, and in foot and leg abnormalities where special shoes and calipers may be needed.

Paediatrics

This department focuses on the care and development of children, and the diseases and ailments that befall them. As paediatrics is concerned with all conditions affecting all systems of the body, a good knowledge of general medical terms and types of investigations is needed. There are many specialists within the paediatric field, such as child endocrinologists, cardiologists, urologists and specialist surgeons.

Since many people are involved in the medical care and general supervision of certain children, copies of letters and reports may have to be sent to a varity of people – the Principal Paediatrician Child Health (PPCH), for example, who works in the Community Services, the community physician, the local health clinic, the general practitioner, the school doctor and health visitor. Children may also be under the care of the psychiatric team, or an educational or clinical psychologist, physiotherapist, speech therapist or dietician. Children are also frequently referred for ear, nose and throat (ENT) opinion.

The paediatric secretary may also be responsible for the typing of the summaries on babies who have been in Special Care Baby Unit (SCBU). Most of these babies are premature and some born at 28 weeks of gestation or earlier need to remain there for a long time and often have a stormy passage before being finally discharged home. Consequently reports tend to be long with much technical detail. In some hospitals typing up these summaries would be the work of the obstetric secretary.

Pathology

This is essentially a laboratory-based department with few specific patients attached to it.

Pathology is the study of disease – in all its aspects. From a clinical point of view, the pathology department is very much concerned with the diagnosis of a disease: it is here that body fluid and tissues samples are sent for microscopic examination, for the culture of organisms and for the testing of sensitivity of organisms to various antibiotics.

Pathology embraces many aspects and the department is divided into several areas of speciality:

- Histopathology and Cytology
- Microbiology
- Chemical pathology (biochemistry)
- Haematology.

Histopathology and Cytology

Histopathology deals with disease processes in tissues and organs; cytology is concerned with actual cell structure.

The consultant histopathologist will report on all the tumours, organs and tissues removed at surgery and also carries out the post-mortem examinations (autopsies). The consultant is usually also a consultant in cytology and examines individual cells looking for abnormal and malignant changes. A large amount of work in cytology is in the examination of cervical smears. Sometimes urine and other body fluids are also sent for cytological examination.

The secretary in the department is actively involved in the typing of histology, cytology and post-mortem reports. This may be typing from handwritten slips, audio tapes, or, less commonly, shorthand. Many departments are computerized to facilitate some of the tasks.

The histology terminology is very specialized, and for post-mortems, knowledge of general medical terminology is necessary. Again, this is a very busy department as specimens from many operations are sent for histological examination. Microscopic examination of tissue during the operation is sometimes carried out (frozen section). This is so that the surgeon does not have to wait several days and can decide whether to proceed to more radical surgery should the biopsy show malignancy. Post-mortems are carried out to determine the cause of death and the post-mortem report will cover all systems of the body and be set out in a fairly standard form. In cases of suspicious, unexplained, violent or sudden death, deaths following some accidents, and surgical operations, an inquest by the coroner has to be held. The coroner commissions the report which is then sent to him. A large number of post-mortems carried out in hospital are coroner's cases – many of them as the result of persons being brought in dead (BID) to Accident and Emergency following collapse or accident.

In addition to the medically qualified, the histology staff will consist of laboratory technicians of all grades and an anatomical pathology technician in charge of the mortuary. The secretary will communicate with all members of staff and with other departments in the hospital. Many telephone calls will be from doctors regarding reports, from the histology unit of other hospitals, and from the coroner's officer. When issuing verbal reports the identify of the caller, and the name, age or date of birth and hospital number of the patient should always be checked. It is important to remember that some of these results profoundly influence the treatment of the patient (for example, whether or not to amputate a limb). To this end, it may be the policy of the hospital or department to allow only medical staff to give results over the telephone so it is important to find this out first.

Microbiology

Microbiology is the science dealing with the study of microorganisms, such as bacteria and viruses. The consultant microbiologist has an important role to play in the control of infection and may be involved in counselling staff looking after AIDS patients.

The laboratory staff send out the result reports. Familiarity with the names of organisms (usually Latin) and antibiotics can soon be achieved. Secretarial duties are confined to the consultant's and other doctors' correspondence; some will be of an urgent nature advising treatment and precautions in regard to serious infections. Other duties are mainly the normal secretarial ones required in running an office and dealing with telephone enquiries.

Chemical pathology (biochemistry)

This is concerned with the chemistry of the body. Tests such as those of liver and thyroid function, and hormone levels are just some of the many which come into this category. These results and those from haematology are usually computerized. The chemical pathologist may share a secretary with one of the other pathologists.

Haematology

This is the study of blood and its disorders. The haematologist treats patients suffering from diseases of the blood such as anaemia, leukaemia and lymphatic disorders and also supervises all tests relating to blood cells. They are also in charge of the blood transfusion service.

The secretarial duties are similar to those of a secretary to any consultant physician or surgeon who sees patients at clinics and admits them under their care to the ward when necessary (see Chapter 2). As well as the usual haematology clinics, anticoagulant clinics are held for patients on anti-coagulants (blood thinners) (see Chapter 8).

Plastic surgery

This speciality is concerned with restorative surgery. Among the patients are those with congenital abnormalities commonly affecting the hand or face, such as absence of thumb or ear, hare-lip or cleft palate. Other patients are those who have received mutilating injuries or burns requiring intricate reconstructive procedures using skin grafts and skin and/or muscle flaps. Another group referred to the plastic surgeon will have had extensive surgery carried out to remove malignant tumours in the area of neck, face, breast and limbs, creating defects which may require skin grafting, rebuilding of structures and perhaps insertion of a prosthesis. The plastic surgeon may also run an outpatient operating session for the removal of small lesions under local anaesthetic.

Only a minor part of the plastic surgeon's work in health service hospitals is devoted to cosmetic surgery. However, some purely cosmetic operations will always be performed to provide the junior surgeons in training with the necessary experience.

Some hospitals have a Burns Unit. The secretary working there should have a good knowledge of common investigations and general medical terminology as often patients are acutely ill suffering lung and kidney complications, as well as septicaemia (blood infection).

The patient's stay in hospital is usually protracted. Burn sites require frequent change of dressings under anaesthetic, and many restorative operations may be necessary using skin grafts to cover the burnt areas. Those patients nursed on ventilators will also be under the care of the anaesthetist.

Psychiatry

The psychiatric department will look after patients with mental disorders of varying severity. In a large general hospital it will probably have a Day Hospital and Drug Dependency Unit as well as clinic facilities and wards for in-patients. The secretary's office may be located in the Day Hospital or near the wards, in which case she will certainly meet patients. A few patients may be in a very disturbed, depressed or even aggressive state and will consequently need sympathetic handling. Some offices have access to an alarm button so that support can be obtained quickly from a qualified member of staff should a threatening situation arise.

There are many conditions needing psychiatric help, such as schizophrenia, personality and behavioural disorders, anxiety states, depressive, manic and obsessional illnesses, anorexia nervosa and addiction to drugs and alcohol.

Often whole families need counselling because of the stress engendered when one member of the family becomes ill in this way. Sometimes illnesses can be caused by attitudes and behaviour within the family itself, making communication and understanding more difficult. Adults and children can have stress-related illnesses which are manifested by physical symptoms and they are usually referred for psychiatric treatment when all conventional medical tests have proved negative and the trouble is felt to be of psychological rather than physical origin.

Psychiatrists may have to deal with child abuse cases and give evidence in court or may be asked to submit a report on the state of mind of a person accused or convicted of serious crime. The duties of the particular psychiatrist will reflect on the type of work the secretary has to undertake.

In general terms, however, most letters and reports are long and in some cases of a distressing nature. Telephone calls need to be handled tactfully and understanding given to patients and relatives. A mature approach is required, and a good standard of written English is more important than specialized terminology.

The department has strong links with the Community Medicine department of the hospital; thus care stretches into the community through psychiatric nurses, social workers, health visitors, child guidance teams, clinical and educational psychologists and many support groups including those looking after the mentally handicapped. The secretary will liaise with many of these as well as with the doctors, nurses and therapists concerned with the patient's treatment in hospital.

Radiotherapy

This is the treatment of (mainly malignant) disease by ionizing radiation (radiology) such as X-rays, beta(β)-rays and gamma(γ)-rays. As expensive and sophisticated equipment is involved, not all hospitals have a radiotherapy unit and so patients may have to be sent to another hospital in the area. However, there is always a consultant radiologist either visiting, or available at another hospital for these referrals. The actual X-ray treatment though, is prescribed by a radiologist (a doctor), is performed by the radiographer.

Oncology is the knowledge and study of tumours and a radiologist usually works closely with oncologists or chemotherapists who supervise the drugs used to treat various cancers.

Renal Medicine

This is a specialist unit concerned with kidney disease.

Rheumatology

This department specializes in the non-surgical care of patients with disease affecting their joints. Rehabilitation forms a large part of the rheumatologist's work as many rheumatic diseases are crippling in nature. The department may also include a Sport's Injury clinic and will have close liaison with the orthopaedic surgeons, referring patients for example, for tendon, cartilage, hip and knee surgery.

It is helpful for the secretary to know the specific terms associated with rheumatology and orthopaedics as well as general medicine.

X-ray/Radiology

In contrast to the radiotherapy department, the radiology department is concerned largely with investigative procedures. The main secretarial duties are typing the reports of X-rays, ultrasound and other examinations. A good knowledge of anatomical terms is required as a report can deal with any part of the body from a fractured skull to a toe. Detecting broken bones, however, is only one part of the use of X-rays. Numerous investigations are undertaken to check the functions of all systems of the body and to look for abnormalities such as tumours, stones, ulcers, and in the case of arteries, narrowing by atheroma (mass of plaque).

Ultrasound ('sonar') scans are widely used these days, especially to examine the pelvis, abdomen and the renal tract. They are used extensively in obstetrics to establish gestation (age of the fetus) by measuring the fetus and to detect some abnormalities. Special scans, some using radioactive isotopes/radionuclides (nuclear medicine) are employed, for example in kidney, thyroid, bone and brain investigations.

Generally, the secretary needs audiotyping skills. In some hospitals however, direct reporting is favoured. If this is the case, the secretary sits at the typewriter in a darkened room with the radiologist who looks at the X-ray films and dictates the findings directly to her to take down. Familiarity with the terminology is especially necessary here, and as X-ray is usually a very busy department, speed and accuracy are of the essence.

There are normally some four or five consultant radiologists in a large hospital as well as several registrars. All carry out complicated investigations and reporting, so the workload is heavy. There may be several part-time secretaries as well as a full-time one. Reports have to be sent out to consultants, wards and to GPs, and the secretary will have other additional administrative duties including maintaining the filing system. There is no patient contact except for seeing the patient in the department if the office is near the waiting area. Contact is mostly with radiologists, radiographers and reception staff. Many telephone calls are from GPs and hospital staff enquiring about results and the identity of the caller should always be checked before giving out a verbal report.

Chapter 2
Secretarial Duties

Some hospitals have a secretarial pool or bureau solely for the workload of all junior doctors; other hospitals have pool secretaries as an additional aid to individual or departmental secretaries. This layer system can be beneficial in giving valuable experience to junior secretaries without their having to take on too much responsibility. Some units have a small team of secretaries headed by a senior secretary whose task is to delegate the work, doing some themself, and taking overall responsibility.

However, the most usual practice is that of one personal secretary with their own office working for one consultant and the associated medical team. This team usually consists of a senior registrar or registrar, senior house officer (SHO) and/or house officer. In some departments there may be a clinical assistant instead of, or as well as, a registrar and unlike the registrar this is a permanent appointment. In a teaching hospital medical students are attached to the team, or 'Firm' as it is often called.

The consultant and their team need the services of a good secretary. The secretary's main role is to assist in the documentation in the patient's medical records (or notes) by typing the letters and summaries containing important information sent to GPs and other doctors concerned in the treatment of the patient. The secretary acts as a liaison between the patient and medical staff, usually by telephone contact and by sorting out problems in regard to appointments, admissions and test results. Although the secretary is not permitted to pass on any medical information to the patient, a helpful and reassuring approach with knowledge of the correct way to answer queries is a valuable service. Confidentiality must, of course, be strictly observed and no information about a patient must be passed on to anyone not concerned with the patient's medical care.

The following are required in the secretary's office, in addition to a good typewriter/word processor, transcriber etc:

- A copy of the hospital internal telephone directory; instructions on how to make outside calls, transferring calls and the bleep system, British Telecom directory and list of numbers relevant to the department.
- A list of local general practitioners, their addresses and telephone numbers.
- The consultants' timetables with telephone numbers where they can be reached and bleep numbers of their team.

- A copy of the *British National Formulary* (BNF) or *MIMS* for drug names and information.
- A good medical dictionary: there should be a large comprehensive one in the department but the secretary may find it useful to have a personal copy. An English dictionary is also helpful.
- A copy of *The Medical Directory*: an independent two-volume publication of the names of most doctors, listed alphabetically. It also contains all the health service hospitals, with details of staff and lists of doctors in local areas.
- A notebook in which to enter receipt and subsequent destination of patients' case notes.
- An adequate supply of stationery and office equipment (all supplied by the hospital), including pads for messages and plenty of pens. It is extremely useful if the secretary has the benefit of the job description left by the previous post-holder as duties in every department vary to a certain extent.

Basic duties

The basic secretarial duties may be summarized as follows:

- Receiving telephone calls and taking appropriate action.
- Opening and sorting mail – unless marked 'Personal' or 'Confidential'.
- Typing outpatient clinic letters.
- Typing discharge summaries.
- Sorting and filing pathology and X-ray results.
- General correspondence.

Telephone calls

The majority of telephone calls are from general practitioners, patients, other doctors, secretaries and Medical Records department. Most calls are concerning appointments, results of tests and whereabouts of patient case notes. The secretary experienced in their consultant's practice and the working of the hospital will be able to deal with most of these queries on their own.

Opening and sorting mail

The post will consist mainly of referral letters from GPs, and letters from other doctors asking for information about a patient. There will also be the internal mail consisting of investigation results, hospital administration information and minutes of meetings. Medical journals and advertising literature will also arrive. These should all be placed in appropriate order for the consultant to see. Referral letters from general practitioners are read by the consultant who indicates if the appointment is urgent or routine. It may be left to the secretary to arrange the appointments either through the appoint-

```
┌─────────────────────────────────────────────────────────────┐
│     Area Health Authority Crest                               │
│     Name of Area Health Authority                             │
│     Name of Hospital                                          │
│   ──────────────────────────────────────────────             │
│                                                               │
│                                    Hospital address:          │
│                                                               │
│                                                               │
│                                    Telephone:                 │
│                                                               │
│                                    Dated: typed               │
│   Date of clinic:                                             │
│                                                               │
│   LMT/RK/3  60  14   (dictating doctor's initials + secretary's initials │
│                       (plus patient's hospital number)        │
│                                                               │
│   GP's name                                                   │
│   Address                                                     │
│                                                               │
│                                                               │
│                                                               │
│   Dear Dr.                                                    │
│   Re: Name of patient + dob (date of birth)                   │
│       Address of patient                                      │
│                                                               │
│                                                               │
│                                                               │
│                                                               │
│                                                               │
│                                                               │
│                                                               │
│   Yours sincerely,                                            │
│                                                               │
│                                                               │
│                                                               │
│   Name of doctor plus qualifications                          │
│   Position held – e.g. Consultant Physician/Surgical Registrar/SHO in │
│             Paediatrics etc.                                  │
└─────────────────────────────────────────────────────────────┘
```

Fig. 2.1 Usual form of clinic letter on headed hospital notepaper.

ment clerks, or if the appointments are on the computer and the secretary has a password to get into the system, the secretary may make or alter appointments directly. When information is asked about a patient from another doctor, the secretary is required to get the case notes from Medical Records. All results of investigations have to be seen and initialled by a doctor (the consultant or registrar) before filing in the patient's notes as further action may be necessary.

Typing outpatient clinic letters

Most patients seen in the outpatient clinics will have a letter dictated to the GP or referring doctor after their visit. The amount of work involved varies according to the size and frequency of the clinics, but it is often considerable. A copy of every letter has to be inserted in the notes and failure to do this can cause serious repercussions. Some consultants require their secretary to type their findings and recommendations into the history sheets of the actual case notes without writing anything themselves. This can present difficulties to an inexperienced secretary not familiar with the terminology as there may be no written notes to follow as a guideline.

Some consultants like their secretary to attend the clinic with them and to take shorthand but it is less common today and the majority of letters are done by audio-typing.

When a patient is seen for the first time in Outpatients it is usual for a large number of tests to be ordered and it is helpful if the secretary can retain the patient's notes, after the letters have been typed. It is best to keep these notes in a special filing cabinet for those awaiting results of investigations.

The letters are normally in a standard form (see Fig. 2.1). The initials of the dictating doctor, the secretary's initials and the patient's record number are at the top. The heading should consist of the patient's name, date of birth (or age), and the patient's address. The letters are written on headed hospital notepaper with an unheaded copy for filing in the notes. The date of dictation and typing is also often shown, as well as the date of the clinic.

Typing discharge summaries

Every patient admitted to hospital has a summary sent to their GP on discharge. A short note handwritten by the house officer is sent immediately the patient leaves the ward to be followed by a fuller summary later (see Fig. 2.2). The notes of patients discharged from the ward are usually sent to the secretary, probably by the ward clerks. It is helpful if the summaries are dictated as soon as possible by the doctor responsible because delays can cause enormous backlogs of both notes and work. If the summary is not dictated and typed promptly the notes may be removed for the patient's out-patient clinic appointment. The summary contains the patient's date of admission, discharge, diagnosis, operations if any, course in hospital, and treatment on discharge. The summary is sent to the patient's GP and a copy is kept in the notes. Some secretaries keep a copy in the office as well, for reference. On completion of the discharge summary the notes go to Hospital Activities Analysis (HAA) recently renamed Hospital Episode Statistics (HES) for coding. Information such as diagnosis, operations and complications are collated by computer to allow analysis of the activities within the hospital. Every patient's notes leaving the secretary's office should be booked out in a special 'booking out' book with name, number, date and destination so that an accurate record is available to help trace the notes later. Failure to do this can cause *hours* of wasted time in searching for notes.

Name of Area Health Authority

Name of hospital

Name of consultant

Patient

DOB

Address

Diagnosis:

Operation:

Hospital no.

Date of admission

Date of discharge

History

Examination

Treatment and progress

Drugs on discharge

Follow up arrangements

Signature
Name of doctor
Position held

Date typed + secretary's initials

Fig. 2.2   One form of hospital summary/discharge letter (often there are printed forms for this).

Sorting and filing pathology and X-ray results

A large number of investigations are ordered for both in- and outpatients. Most of the results eventually end up in the secretary's office. All results should be shown to a doctor first, but many results come from the ward after the patient has been discharged and the notes are gone – and since these have already been seen and initialled they require filing only. This can be a daunting task because of the number of results and the difficulty in tracing the notes. A regular trip to Medical Records for this purpose is paramount if the situation is to be kept under control.

A list of patients attending current outpatient clinics of each consultant is sent to their secretary. This allows the secretary to sort and send all the results for patients who are attending the clinic to be available for the doctors. If this is not done a great deal of time can be wasted with the clinic ringing up for results which should be in the notes. The secretary can help a lot to ensure this does not happen.

General correspondence

In every department there is always a certain amount of general correspondence to be dealt with in addition to that already described.

Additional duties

The secretary is responsible for the organization and smooth running of the office so that information and case notes are readily available. Stationery should be in good supply and office equipment in working order. Every hospital has a slightly different method of ordering and repair so the secretary should become familiar with this as soon as possible.

In every department there is usually a visual display unit (VDU) or computer to look up patient's details, and after instruction the secretary will probably have a password to get into the appointment system and other facilities. Most departments also have access to a photocopier.

In addition to the basic duties outlined some secretaries may be required to do some of the following tasks:

- Arrange meetings (e.g. committee, department, or with drug representatives).
- Organize catering for some meetings.
- Take minutes at meetings.
- Arrange doctors' locum cover (normally done in liaison with Personnel).
- Draw up on-call rotas.
- Keep the consultant's diary and arrange commitments outside the hospital.
- Organize transport for patients attending Outpatients by contacting the transport officer as soon as possible. The transport officer usually has an office in the area of Outpatient Appointments or Accident and Emergency.

- Organize domiciliary visits by the consultant to the patient's home. A special form needs to be filled in for this purpose.
- Arrange minor operation sessions, i.e. organize the List in advance; send for patients giving them information such as time, date, place of admission and the importance of no food or drink (as appropriate). Type up list and distribute. The waiting list may also be kept by some secretaries.
- Collect relevant information for solicitors' reports and Criminal Injuries Board enquiries.
- Type papers and lectures for medical staff and liaise with the photographic department in respect of slides and projectors for meetings, and teaching.

Chapter 3
Medical Records, Appointments and Admissions: Departments and Procedures

Medical Records

Medical Records is an important department whose function is the storage of patients' case notes and the retrieval or 'pulling' of these notes for out-patient clinics, admission to hospital, medicolegal enquiries and other reasons. In charge is the medical records manager whose duties are wide ranging.

The medical secretaries come under the jurisdiction of the medical records manager and their budget – as do the clerical and reception staff of Medical Records, Appointments, Admissions, Accident and Emergency and Out-patients. To help with these responsibilities there is usually a supervisor/manager for Secretarial Services, Admissions and Outpatients, as well as a deputy medical records manager, but in some large hospitals, staff may be divided into service centres by specialities or groups of specialities and then there would be no senior medical secretary or deputy medical records officer.

Filing, storage and retrieval of notes

Hospitals vary in the system used for filing case notes but generally it is numerical rather than alphabetical, the latter only used in small indices in the hospital, such as casualty cards.

The most usual combination for filing is the six digit system. For example to retrieve Mrs Smith's case notes, number 28 45 63:

Find row 63
Look for the 45s
Then look for number 28

New notes are added to the beginning of every sequence from 01 00 01 to 01 99 99 for example after the 28s, then 29 and 30 and so on. This allows for a large number of new notes to be added to the existing system. Some hospitals may use forward numerical filing starting from 1–999999, then starting again with A in front of the figures, then B and so on.

Terminal six digit filing may also be used. Then, to find case notes number 316204, go to:

Section 4 – 000004 (sections 0 – 9)

Row 20   – 000204 (row or shelves 00, 01 etc. – 99)
Then 16s – 016204 (order 00, 01 etc. – 99)
Then 3   – 316204 (order 0 – 9)

Although this system does makes mis-filed notes extremely difficult to find, the advantage is that the system can be used with other methods by adding noughts to make six digits should a separate system be required for, say, patients attending in the last two or three years.

Colour coding is often used with all these systems to help prevent mis-filing and to make it easier to find a 'lost' file. The colour code may relate to individual consultants or to specialities.

Storage space for notes is a problem in all hospitals making for compromise rather than ideal arrangements. Some notes are destroyed – with the consultant's approval – after a number of years but there are many exceptions to this, such as paediatric patients, cancer registry patients, and research projects, all of which have to be kept for much longer. Some hospitals use microfiche and microfilm notes. This creates extra space but demands special equipment and a person employed to do the micro-filming, and retrieval when the notes are required.

It is usual practice for the notes of patients not attending for many years to be kept in separate storage areas, such as disused wards or basement rooms. The notes of deceased patients are also stored outside the main system. Very thick notes may be divided into separate folders and kept on specially marked shelves.

Medical Records' clerical staff 'pull' the notes of all patients who are on the current appointment list for a consultant's outpatient clinic. Individual clerks are allocated responsibility for a particular consultant's list and it is their job also to ensure that the X-rays are also available when the patient attends the clinic, although sometimes the X-ray department staff are responsible for this. It may also be the duty of a member of the Medical Records staff to prepare the notes seeing that all investigation results are available and that the notes are in proper order. New patients are issued with case note folders by the appointment clerks. It is now normal practice for the main patient index to be computerized so it is easy to find out via the visual display unit (VDU) if the patient has attended the hospital before.

Difficulties can arise when the patient's notes are not in Medical Records. Every set of notes has a tracer, normally in the notes or left in place of the notes when they have been removed. This tracer should contain the information of (1) where the notes are being taken to, and (2) the date they are removed and preferably the signature or initials of the person removing them.

If the patient has attended an outpatient clinic recently or has been admitted, the secretary often has the notes for letters, results or discharge summaries. Therefore, secretaries receive many calls and queries from Medical Records regarding the whereabouts of notes. The secretary will have many occasions to go to Medical Records for notes or for filing purposes and it is worth emphasizing that no notes should be taken without the tracer being filled in legibly as to the notes' destination. So much distress is caused by missing notes that every effort must be made to prevent this occurrence.

Appointments

A GP will refer a patient to hospital to see a particular consultant by letter. This letter can be taken to the Appointments Desk by hand or sent by post. Appointments are not normally given over the telephone except in cases of a patient cancelling an appointment and wanting to make another, or a long-standing patient requiring follow-up appointments. The telephone is best avoided because of the volume of calls received and the difficulty in getting through, and if no appointment can be given, it is of course very frustrating.

Most consultants see all their referral letters, marking them urgent or routine so that the appointment clerks know when to make the appointment for. A few spaces are left on every clinic for urgent referrals but they can be quickly filled and it is often left to the secretary to put in any 'late' patients on the consultant's clinic.

Some patients fail to attend appointments (FTA or DNA for 'did not attend'). Depending on the circumstances patients are either sent another appointment, or the GP informed or the notes returned to Medical Records without any action being taken. Most doctors like to see the notes of those failing to attend to decide on the appropriate action.

Admissions

Organizing admission to hospital may still be one of the duties of the medical secretary (under the direction of the consultant or registrar) but it is becoming increasingly rare in most hospitals. Normally there is a central Admissions Office where the waiting lists are held. Patients will be on the routine or urgent waiting lists according to their conditions. Emergency cases are admitted directly from Accident and Emergency.

If the patient is to be admitted, the doctor doing the outpatient clinic will fill in an admission card with the details, and usually the nursing staff or secretary, see that these cards go to the Admissions Office. In some departments a diary is used so that the patient can be given the date for admission there-and-then in the clinic. In urgent cases, patients may be admitted directly from the clinic. At clinics outside the hospital, the admission cards are usually given to the secretary by the doctor on their return so that the necessary procedures can be instituted. Most patients on waiting lists are waiting for an operation. There is not usually a waiting list for medical admissions.

Every week the registrar of a 'Firm' together with the Admissions Office (or secretary, if in their brief), lists the names of the patients to come in (TCI). A letter is then sent to the patient with details and instructions.

Patients for admission are usually asked to ring the ward or Admissions

Office on the morning of admission to make certain that a bed is still free as emergency admissions can alter the bed availability. It is therefore very important to let the Admissions Office and the registrar concerned know if a patient cancels an admission, so that another patient can be asked to come in. The ward should also be informed if the cancelled admission is for that day.

A secretary may have several calls from patients regarding admissions, especially about the length of time on the waiting list. It is very important to ascertain that the patient is definitely on the waiting list as mistakes can occur. Normally a GP will ask to speak to the consultant or registrar personally if a patient's condition warrants an early admission. Thus, if a patient is very anxious they should be instructed to see their GP. In cases where the GP cannot be contacted and the patient is very worried about some present disturbing symptom they can be advised to attend Accident and Emergency – or dial 999 if the situation worsens dramatically.

Chapter 4
Hospital Administration and Staff

This chapter briefly outlines the role of some other members of the hospital staff whose jobs and skills are totally different but should be known by, or, are particularly relevant to the secretary's work.

Administration

The management of hospitals is undergoing change. Hitherto District General Hospitals have been run by the Local Health Authority and this Authority was usually divided into two Units, the Acute Unit and the Community Unit, together forming the District. As a result of health service reforms an increasing number of NHS hospitals are becoming self-governing health service Trusts.

Directly Managed Units

These units remain under Local Health Authority control and are found in districts where NHS Trusts have not yet been established.

The unit general manager (Acute Services) is in charge of the administration of the hospital. To help there would probably be an operational manager, a deputy operational manager and operational administrators and assistant administrators. The senior administrators hold budgets and have special responsibility for various departments in the hospital. Money for equipment, buildings, extra staff etc. has to be sanctioned by the administrators in consultation with interested parties. Thus, a great deal of their work is involved in committees, planning future expenditure and policies, as well as in devising means of cutting costs and increasing efficiency.

The medical secretary will soon get to know those administrators especially relevant to their consultant, and will probably have many occasions on which to type letters to the unit or operational managers. The deputy operational manager may be the person who deals with all complaints from patients and the medicolegal aspect.

The Medical Records manager is in close touch with the operational manager – normally being responsible directly to them.

The Community Unit also has equivalent administrative staff led by a unit general manager (Community Services).

The District is headed by the chairman of the Area Health Authority, and the District general manager is senior to the two Unit General Managers (Acute and Community). There are District managers for finance, technical services, estates and personnel etc. These managers are probably housed outside the hospital in District Headquarters, although some hospitals have facilities for District Headquarters within the hospital confines.

NHS Trusts

A Trust Board, with a chairman and executive and non-executive members, is different from a directly managed unit in that it is responsible directly to the Department of Health for the running of the hospital. The Trust is responsible for providing health services which are contracted and paid for by a variety of purchasing authorities.

The chief executive officer of the Trust is equivalent to the managing director and included among the executive directors there will be a senior consultant as medical director and also a director of nursing.

Occupational Health

All applicants for permanent positions within the Health Authority have to be passed fit by Occupational Health before being appointed. They may be required to fill in a questionnaire only or they may be asked to have a chest X-ray, blood test, or if there are any queries about their health, to see the doctor. A local GP may be the doctor appointed to Occupational Health. Staff who have had long absences because of sickness may be requested to see the doctor to assess their suitability on health grounds for continuing in their post.

Depending on the facilities in the particular department, staff taken ill at work may be able to see the occupational health nurse, lie down for a while, and perhaps consult the doctor.

Preventive medicine forms a large part of the role of Occupational Health and the nurse in charge may give talks on such subjects as diet, smoking, exercise and general healthy living. Information and leaflets on all aspects of health care can be obtained from Occupational Health.

Postgraduate medical centre

Most district hospitals have a Postgraduate Medical Centre with a library, lecture theatre and perhaps restaurant facilities for the medical staff. Discussion groups, films and lectures are held regularly and there is usually valuable liaison between local GPs and consultant staff on these occasions. A clinical tutor, administrator/secretary and librarian, form some of the staff of the Centre. The library facilities may be particularly helpful for doctors studying for examinations or writing papers.

Medical staff

Consultants

The consultant is a fully qualified doctor who has then gone on to study and specialize in a certain field (e.g. rheumatology). A consultant may be employed full-time at one hospital, may work part-time for the health service and part-time privately, or may be employed in different health service hospitals. Most health service consultants practise privately in their non-health service time.

The consultant heads a team of doctors, the most junior of whom is their house officer.

Junior house officers

After five to six years' full-time study, the medical student, on passing his final exams, qualifies as a 'doctor'. However, this is just the beginning of many years' postgraduate study and training, and 'working up the ladder' – starting with one year's house jobs (six months of medicine and six months of surgery) before full registration as a doctor.

This pre-registration year is very taxing and the doctor may be 'on-call' every two-to-three nights. The doctor 'lives in' at the hospital. The house officer (HO) is the doctor the medical secretary may see most of.

Senior house officers

The house officer's immediate senior (usually 1–3 years post-registration) is the senior house officer (SHO). This grade is usually for two or five years, and so some SHOs may be quite experienced. Most SHO posts are part of 'rotations' of four to six six-month posts giving the 'junior' doctor (as all doctors below consultant are referred to) a wide range of experience within general and more specific areas of medicine or surgery.

Registrars

Registrars are usually committed to one field of medicine or surgery (e.g. paediatrics or orthopaedics). After two or three years the registrar becomes a senior registrar (SR) who is the most experienced of the 'junior' doctors. Registrar and senior registrar training is arranged in rotations of six- to twelve-month posts in one or several hospitals.

Qualifications

All doctors have a basic medical degree such as MB or BS (Bachelor of Medicine, Bachelor of Surgery).

Most specialists have specialist qualifications attaching them to one of the Royal Colleges. These special 'membership' or 'fellowship' examinations are taken in two or three parts over several years. The final possession of these qualifications is usually achieved in registrar and senior registrar grades.

The following is a selection of these qualifications, a full list may be found at the front of *The Medical Directory*.

Examples:
(All are of equal status)

FFARCS	Fellow of the Faculty of Anaesthetists, Royal College of Surgeons.
FRCR	Fellow of the Royal College of Radiologists.
FRCS	Fellow of the Royal College of Surgeons. Most senior registrars and consultants hold the FRCS. Once doctors becomes FRCS they are commonly known as 'Mr/Mrs/Miss' to indicate that they are surgeons as opposed to physicians.
FRCS Glas/Ed/or I	Indicates that the surgeon is a Fellow of the Royal College of Surgeons of Glasgow, Edinburgh or Ireland.
FRCS Orth	This is an additional orthopaedic fellowship.
MRCP	These letters after a doctor's name denote a member of the Royal College of Physicians. This is of equal status to the surgical fellowship (FRCS) and is held by senior registrars and consultants in medical specialities.
MRCOG	Member of the Royal College of Obstetricians and Gynaecologists.
MRCPath	Member of the Royal College of Pathologists.
MRCPsych	Member of the Royal College of Psychiatrists.

Many doctors have additional qualifications (e.g. an MSc) and should be asked how they like to have their letters signed.

Nursing staff

The system of nurse education is undergoing a period of change. In 1988 Project 2000 was introduced to prepare the nursing profession to meet the changing health care needs of the population. The course lasts three years and successful completion will lead to qualification and registration of only one level of nurse for which the title Registered Nurse (RN) is to be used. From September 1993 the United Kingdom Central Council for Nursing, Midwifery and Health Visiting (UKCC) register will clearly show the levels and designations of each nurse but recognizes that some nurses may wish to continue to use their existing titles. The register will be divided into 15 parts to take into account the various qualifications.

Those who qualified before the introduction of Project 2000 may use different titles. Nurses were previously designated on the UKCC register as either first level nurses, using the title Registered General Nurse (RGN) equivalent to the former State Registered Nurse (SRN), or second level nurses using the title Enrolled Nurse (EN) equivalent to the former State Enrolled Nurse (SEN).

The clinical grading structure and salaries of nurses start from grade A or B for nursing auxiliaries and support workers and proceed upwards from C, D, E, F, G, H to I, depending on qualifications, experience and post held.

The Nursing Administration Department plays a vital part in organizing nursing cover throughout the hospital. In charge is the Director of Nursing Services, equivalent to the Matron of former times. Below this are nurse managers of different grades, charge nurses or ward sisters, staff nurses, student nurses in training, and the non-qualified auxiliary nurses/support workers – plus also the ward clerks, although in some hospitals the ward clerks may be members of the Medical Records department.

As the consultant surgeon or physician will have their own ward, or beds in a particular ward, the secretary will get to know the permanent nursing staff and ward clerks attached to that ward.

Professions allied to medicine

Working within the hospital setting are a range of health care professions, such as chiropody, orthoptics, dietetics, and a range of therapies, radiography, occupational therapy and physiotherapy. The medical secretary needs to be familiar with a number of these groups and their role. Outlined below are some examples; these have been listed alphabetically for ease of reference.

Chiropodists

Chiropodists look after patients' feet particularly elderly and diabetic patients who are susceptible to suffering from circulatory problems. Hospitals may have their own chiropodist or access to a visiting chiropodist, who may hold clinics on a regular basis.

Dietitians

The dietitian sees patients referred by the medical or nursing staff and provides dietary advice for those with conditions such as obesity, food allergies, kidney disease and diabetes. The dietitian will also provide advice on how to achieve a balanced diet to avoid ill health.

Occupational therapists

Occupational therapists work mainly with the physically and mentally handicapped and the mentally ill. The aim is rehabilitation to enable people with problems, both temporary and permanent, to cope with everyday life.

The occupational therapist may provide therapy for inpatients or day patients in creative activities such as painting, carpentry, dressmaking and cookery. Some occupational therapy departments are equipped with a kitchen so that patients can learn new skills or relearn old skills to help them to cope at home. The occupational therapist may visit a patient's home to identify what aids are required for activities such as bathing. The safety of the home environment is assessed and according to the individual needs of the patient, aids and alterations to the home are recommended.

Orthoptics

Orthoptics are mainly concerned with the diagnosis and treatment of squint and other disorders of binocular vision and eye movement. Many of the patients are young and orthoptists work closely with paediatricians in the assessment and care of the handicapped child. They also see patients referred by the neurologist, neurosurgeon and physician.

Pharmacists

Every hospital has a pharmacy department with a dispensary for inpatient and outpatient drugs. In charge is the principal pharmacist and there is always someone responsible for providing drug information.

Physiotherapists

Physiotherapists treat all kinds of injury and disease, and all ages of patient. Physiotherapy is the use of physical means to prevent injury and disease and assist the process of rehabilitation by developing and restoring the function of the body to enable the patient to return to an active and independent life as possible.

Physiotherapists work in hospitals, treating both inpatients and outpatients. They also work in the community, in patients' own homes, in rehabilitation centres and sports centres. Working within the hospital physiotherapy department are receptionists, secretaries and clerical staff.

Radiographers

Radiographers are either diagnostic radiographers or therapeutic radiographers. Diagnostic radiographers are concerned with the diagnostic use of X-rays. They take pictures of suspected damaged areas. A diagnostic radiographer will determine the angle from which the film is to be taken, and process it to allow the radiologist to make a diagnosis. Although this group work mainly in X-ray departments, some examinations may take place on the wards and in operating theatres. Most hospitals maintain 24-hour emergency services for accidents and the radiographer may therefore be required to work occasional night shifts.

Therapeutic radiographers are concerned with radiotherapy treatment as prescribed by a radiologist.

Social workers

Teams of social workers are responsible for patients under various specialities such as medicine, surgery, paediatrics and psychiatry. The social workers perform the normal social services function in relation to illness, home conditions, disability and other benefits, home helps and convalescent facilities. There is a central office situated within the hospital that is open to patients and/or relatives at set times each day.

Speech therapists

Speech therapists help individuals to overcome speech and language problems. A hospital may have one or two qualified speech therapists whose duties may extend to outside clinics and schools. Some of their work is concerned with the young whose speech impediments may include poor pronunciation and stammering or inadequate and immature vocabulary. Other referrals may be as a result of surgical intervention or following nervous system injuries.

Ancillary staff

There are many skilled individuals working in the hospital setting whose support is essential to the smooth running of the hospital. Some examples, listed in alphabetical order are given below.

Audiologists

Audiologists specialize in treating individuals with impaired hearing. People may be referred by the consultant or GP. Those requiring hearing aids may attend for advice, repairs to the aid, and for new batteries. Senior citizens may have a hearing test performed without a consultant or GP referral.

Clinical measurement technicians

These staff perform mainly lung function tests and urodynamic studies. Patients are referred by consultants for these tests in lung conditions, perhaps before operation, and bladder problems such as stress incontinence or frequency. Patients in Intensive Care also require these services.

Electrocardiogram (ECG) technicians

ECG technicians carry out tests using an electrocardiogram (ECG) to assess the function of the heart. This may aid the diagnosis of heart disease or may be prior to surgery. Exercise ECGs are also performed on some patients. Interpretation of the ECG trace is highly skilled and will be seen by a doctor. A copy of the ECG will go into the patient's notes.

Electroencephalogram (EEG) technicians

EEG technicians perform tests using an electroencephalogram (EEG) to measure the activity of the brain. Many patients are those suffering from epilepsy of one kind or another, but some may have brain tumours. Inter-pretation of the EEG trace is highly skilled and will be undertaken by a doctor. A copy will go into the patient's notes.

Medical photographer

Slides and films are taken mostly of patients undergoing surgical procedures, pre- and post-operatively, or those with skin conditions, rare tumours and congenital abnormalities. The secretary sometimes has to obtain slides from the photographic department for the consultant's lectures.

Orthotics

Orthotists make and fit orthopaedic appliances. Patients are referred by a hospital consultant.

Plaster technicians

Plaster technicians apply plaster casts, usually in the case of fractures or following corrective surgery. The plaster technician works in close associ-ation with the orthopaedic department, and many patients on return visits to the consultant have their plaster of Paris (POP) removed by the technician before seeing the consultant.

Support staff

In addition to the groups mentioned previously, there are numerous other departments and support staff who contribute towards the day to day running of the hospital. The hospital medical secretary may not come across all those mentioned but it is important to be aware of the existence of such services.

Central Sterile Supplies Department (CSSD)

All syringes, needles, instruments and dressings are sterilized by autoclave and packed in this department. The secretary would only be involved to a lesser degree if the autoclaves break down and operating lists and admissions have to be cancelled.

District fire officer

Every hospital has the services of a district fire and safety officer. Lectures, demonstrations and films are held on a regular basis for hospital staff so that everyone knows what to do in the event of a fire.

Domestic supervisor

The domestic services department deals with the cleaning of the hospital and is run by the domestic supervisor. Any complaints regarding this service should be directed to the supervisor.

Hospital chaplain

A chaplain is appointed to the hospital and holds regular services for patients and staff in the hospital chapel, and visits patients on the wards. There are visiting ministers of most denominations and a list of patients and their religion is available for the chaplain's use.

Information services manager

This manager is in charge of seeing that correct information is fed into the hospital's computer so that bed availability, admission lists, discharges, ward lists, operating lists and other details are readily accessible. Statistics can be obtained on a regular basis – for example, on the number of operations or clinic attendance of an individual consultant. The information systems manager is also concerned with any difficulties with the computer system and for instructing those who need passwords to get into the system for their particular jobs. The sophistication of the information technology systems within hospitals varies considerably.

Personnel

The Personnel department provides staff for the hospital, advertises vacancies, interviews applicants, assesses posts for upgrading, advises on scales of pay and conditions, issues contracts and keeps personal files of permanent staff.

The personnel officer is directly responsible for medical staffing, arranges locum cover and liaises with the accommodation officer.

Porters

Every hospital has a team of porters, headed by a head porter and deputy. Their duties are mainly those of conveying patients by chair or stretcher to other departments within the hospital, moving furniture and equipment, transporting case notes on a regular basis from wards and offices, and collecting and delivering post. Porters may also man the 'Enquiries Desk' and the main entrances. They usually hold keys to most departments and perform certain security functions. They work a shift system so that some are always available.

The head porter is normally extremely knowledgeable about all parts of the hospital and can often help to locate an unused filing cabinet or other equipment the secretary may need.

Theatre porters (or orderlies) perform the task of conveying patients to and from operating theatres. As they are required to go into the theatres they wear the special shoes, caps and gowns worn by the theatre staff.

Relatives officer

The relatives officer is responsible for seeing the relatives of deceased patients, handing over any belongings and ensuring that the correct paperwork is instituted, by doctors and next of kin. They need regular contact with the Coroner's Officer and morticians. In some hospitals they may be called patients' affairs officer or a similar title.

Transport officers

A clerical officer is usually responsible for organizing transport for patients attending hospital. Secretaries often have to initiate this and adequate warning must be given to the transport officer when this is required. An ambulance liaison officer is attached to the hospital and may have an office there. If patients are not disabled, the hospital car service, a voluntary organization, may be able to help.

Voluntary workers – League of Friends

The Friends of a hospital help to raise money to provide extra comforts and amenities for inpatients. They usually run the hospital shop and they or other volunteers look after the patients' library, take the trolley shop around the wards and may read to, or write letters for inpatients. There is usually a voluntary service coordinator on the hospital staff and voluntary help may be used also for patient transport, reception or clerical duties.

Works department

Working in the hospital are a number of people whose services may be required from time to time, such as carpenters, plumbers and electricians.

Part II
Medical Basics

Chapter 5
Body Structures and Functions

The body is conventionally subdivided into systems dealing with particular organs and functions. For example, the cardiovascular system is concerned with the heart and blood vessels, and a cardiologist would be a specialist in diseases and malfunctions of this system.

Some knowledge of the major organ systems of the body is required by the medical secretary, and it will be seen in the chapters following, that many diseases, and the drugs used to treat them, affect a particular system (sometimes others, too). This also applies to the signs and symptoms of the disease, and therefore medical examinations are performed in a systematic way and the subsequent doctor's report, typed by the secretary, will illustrate this.

Depending on the department the secretary may need to know more detail about a particular system, for example the skeletal system in orthopaedics or the female reproductive system in gynaecology.

This chapter contains simple descriptions of the structures and function of each major system of the body. Also included are basic outlines of the ear, nose and throat 'system', and of the eye. These are both surgical specialities examined in more detail in later chapters, but it is fitting that their structural and functional aspects should be considered here. Only dental anatomy is covered later (in Chapter 18 on Oral Surgery and Dentistry). These descriptions are not meant to be comprehensive but should give an idea about the various organs and tissues that are dealt with.

The organ systems of the body comprise the:

- *Skeletal system*   Bones, joints, muscles and tendons. Collectively, these components provide the supporting framework for the organs and soft tissues.
- *Skin*   Tough, supple membrane covering the entire surface of the body. It is also the largest organ in the body.
- *Central nervous system*   Brain and spinal cord. Controls and co-ordinates all body functions and processes. Networks information to and from the peripheral nervous system.
- *Peripheral nervous system*   Nerves outside the central nervous system. Transmits information to the brain (via the spine) and executes instructions from the brain.
- *Cardiovascular system*   Heart and blood vessels. Delivers blood, nutri-

ents, and other essentials to the cells and removes waste products. Functions in association with the respiratory system.

- *Respiratory system*   Air passages and lungs. Ventilates the body and allows the exchange of oxygen and carbon dioxide (waste gas).
- *Gastrointestinal system*   Digestive tract – comprising mouth, oesophagus, stomach, small and large intestines. The liver, gall bladder, biliary duct system and pancreas are accessory organs. Transforms and conveys nutrients and other essentials derived from ingested food to body cells, and collects waste products.
- *Endocrine system*   Hypothalamus and pituitary gland plus reproductive glands, thyroid, parathyroids, adrenal glands, and part of the pancreas. Concerned with the production and regulation of the body's chemical messengers (hormones).
- *Genitourinary system*   Kidneys, ureters, urethra, and reproductive organs. Responsible for water and salts (electrolytes) balance in the body.
- *Lymphatic system*   Lymph ducts and glands, and the spleen. Concerned with the maintenance of the body's tissue fluid environment, the absorption of fat and the defence of the body against invasion by foreign material, e.g. bacteria.
- *Reticuloendothelial system*   Cells present within the body concerned with the removal of particles of foreign matter. Also responsible for removing worn-out red blood cells.
- *Immune system*   A biochemical complex that protects the body from dangerous and foreign organisms. Listed here for completion only.

The skeletal system

The skeletal system comprises the:

- bones
- joints
- muscles
- tendons.

Skull

The bones of the skull are arranged in two parts, the cranium and facial skeleton (see Fig. 5.1).

Cranium

The cranium is made up of eight bones. The upper surface of the cavity is the vault and the lower is the base. The eight bones are named:

- occiput (1)
- parietal (2)
- frontal (1)
- temporal (2)
- sphenoid (1)
- ethmoid (1)   situated at the roof of the nose between the orbits.

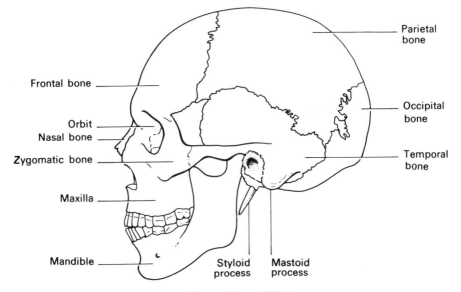

Fig. 5.1 The skull from the side. (*Source* Gibson 1981.)

The line of union adjoining these bones are called sutures. The principal ones are coronal, between the frontal bone and parietal bones, sagittal, between the two parietal bones, and lambdoidal, between the upper borders of the occipital bone and parietal bones.

The facial skeleton
The facial skeleton is made up of 14 bones. These are named:

- nasal (2)   forming the bridge of the nose.
- palate (2)
- lacrimal (2)   forming tear duct and inner angle of the eye.
- malar (2)   the cheek bones which unite to form the zygomatic arch, also known as the zygomatic bones.
- inferior turbinate (2)   outer wall of the nasal fossae.
- vomer (1)   forms the lower part of the bony partition in the nose.
- maxilla (2)   upper jaw.
- mandible (1)   lower jaw – the only moveable bone in the skull.

Chest

The chest (thorax) is a cone-shaped cavity formed by the 12 thoracic vertebrae at the back, the breastbone (sternum) in front, and 12 pairs of ribs at the side.

Below the chest is the diaphragm and above is the root of the neck.

Ribs

There are 12 pairs of ribs, most attached to the breastbone by the costal cartilages. The last two ribs are unattached in front and are called 'floating' ribs.

Between the ribs lie the intercostal muscles.

Spinal column

The spinal (vertebral) column is a flexible structure formed by a number of bones also called vertebrae. Between the bones are pads of tissue called intervertebral discs.

There are 33 vertebral bones. These are named:

- cervical (7)   forming the neck.
- thoracic (12)   forming the back of the thorax or chest.
- lumbar (5)   forming the lumbar region or loins.
- sacral   forming the sacrum.
- coccygeal   forming the coccyx or tail.

When typing reports about the vertebrae they are usually known by the first letter, for example: second cervical vertebra C2; seventh thoracic vertebra T7; but some doctors refer to dorsal vertebrae which are equivalent of thoracic vertebrae.

The intervertebral discs are referred to by the vertebrae above and below, for example: L 4/5 disc.

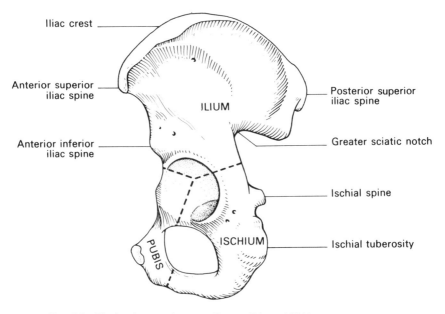

Fig. 5.2   The hip bone, side view. (*Source* Gibson 1981.)

Pelvis

The pelvis made up of four bones. These are named the:

- innominate (2)   the hip bone consisting of the iliac bone (ilium), ischial bone (ischium) and pubic bone
- sacrum
- coccyx.

The hip bone (see Fig. 5.2) is in the front and at the sides with the sacrum and coccyx behind.

Skeleton of the upper limbs

The skeleton of the upper limbs is attached to the skeleton of the trunk by means of the shoulder girdle. This consists of the:

- clavicle
- scapula
- humerus.

The *clavicle* is the collar bone.

The *scapula* (see Fig. 5.3) forms the posterior part of the shoulder girdle. Parts of the scapula commonly mentioned in the typing of reports are the:

acromion process
glenoid cavity
coracoid process.

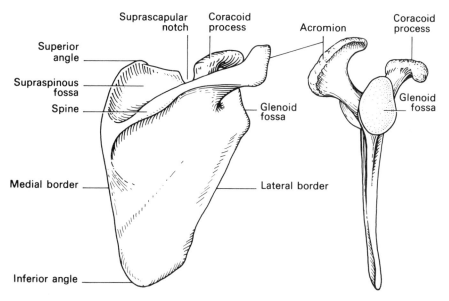

Fig. 5.3   The scapula from the back (left) and side (right) (*Source* Gibson 1981.)

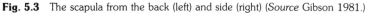

(Scapula is the noun and scapular the adjective.)

The *humerus* is the longest bone of the upper limb. The shoulder joint consists of the humeral head articulating with the glenoid cavity of the scapula.

The humerus has:

- bicipital groove   in which the tendons of the biceps muscle lie, and the spiral or radial groove which gives passage to the radial nerve.
- coronoid fossa   into which the coronoid process of the ulna is received when the elbow is bent fully.
- olecranon fossa   which receives the olecranon process of the ulna when the elbow is completely straight.

The bones of the forearm

These comprise the:

- ulna (1)   the innermost bone.
- radius (1)   the outermost and shorter bone.

(Ulna is the noun and ulnar the adjective.)

The bones of the wrist and hand

These are arranged in groups of the bones:

- carpus   eight bones forming the wrist.
- metacarpals   five bones forming the palm of the hand.
- phalanges   three bones forming the fingers (singular is phalanx) – also the name for bones of the toes. There are only two phalanges in the thumb.

Skeleton of the lower limbs

The bones of the leg consist of the:

- femur; greater trochanter, lesser trochanter
- kneecap (patella)
- tibia
- fibula.

The *femur* is the longest bone in the body. It articulates with the acetabulum (of the pelvis) forming the hip joint. It has a spherical head on the end of the offset neck.

The *greater trochanter* lies where the neck of femur joins the shaft and gives attachment to several muscles including the gluteal muscles.

The *lesser trochanter* gives insertion to the iliopsoas muscle.

The *knee cap (patella)* is a sesamoid bone, that is a bone embedded in a tendon or joint capsule. (Patellar is the adjective referring to the patella.)

The knee joint is a complex hinge joint and contains many important structures such as:

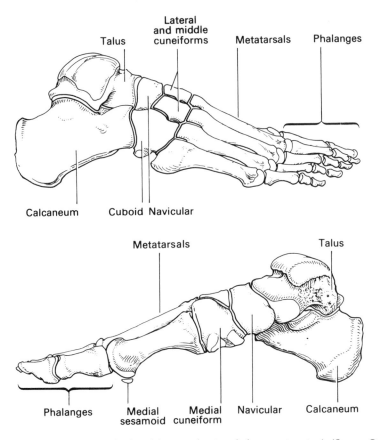

Fig. 5.4   The bones of the foot (above: side view; below: centre view). (*Source* Gibson 1981.)

suprapatellar and prepatellar bursae
anterior and posterior cruciate ligaments
synovial membrane – secreting a lubricating fluid
medial and lateral menisci (often referred to as cartilages).

The *tibia* or shin bone consists of an upper end – the tibial plateau – the shaft, and a lower end. The lower end of the tibia forms part of the ankle joint and is prolonged downwards as the medial *malleolus*.

The *fibula* is the outer and smaller of the two bones below the knee. (Fibular is the adjective referring to the fibula, e.g. he has a fibular fracture.)

The bones of the foot

Three groups of bones (see Fig. 5.4) make up the foot:

* tarsals (7)   these support the weight of the body standing and are the:
  os calcis or calcaneum

    talus
    navicular
    cuboid
    cuneiform (3)
* metatarsals (5)
* phalanges   the big toe has two and the others three.

The skin

The skin is the largest organ in the body and is the body's first line of defence against foreign organisms. The skin covers the body and is divided into two main layers:

* epidermis
* dermis or corium.

Epidermis

The epidermis is composed of stratified epithelium and consists of five layers of cells. From within out, these are the: basal layer, prickle-cell or spinous layer, granular layer, clear layer and horny layer (cuticle). It does not contain any blood vessels. The ducts of the sweat glands pass through it and it also accommodates the hairs. The surface of the epidermis is marked by ridges and lines corresponding to the papillae of the dermis below.

Dermis

The dermis consists of a dense bed of vascular tissue. The nerve endings (tactile bodies) lie in the dermis and also coiled tubes of numerous sweat glands.

Sebaceous glands

Sebaceous glands are found in the skin and open into a hair follicle. They are most numerous in the scalp and face. The glands and ducts are lined by epithelial cells and changes in the cells result in the secretion of sebum. The hair, nails and sebaceous glands are looked upon as appendages of the skin. The part of the hair which projects from the surface is the hair shaft. The amount of pigment in the epidermis dictates the colour of the hair. Associated with the hair follicles are minute involuntary muscles the arrectores pilorum or 'raisers of the hair'.

Nails

Nails are composed of modified skin and lie on nail beds in which the dermis is arranged in ridges. The white part of the nail is called the lunula and is the portion from which the nail grows. The body of the nail is attached to the nail bed and the distal extremity is free. At each side the nail is bounded by a fold of skin termed the nail wall.

The central nervous system

The central nervous system (CNS) comprises the:

- brain
- spinal cord.

The brain and spinal cord are surrounded by the meninges which are a membrane covering. There are also special cranial nerves and arteries.

Brain

The brain is part of the nervous system and is contained within the skull or cranium. The brain consists of the:

- cerebrum
- brainstem
- cerebellum.

The *cerebrum* controls all voluntary movement, tactile sense, the higher centres for speech, intellect, memory, consciousness and the special senses. The *cortex* is an outer covering of grey cells several layers deep, lying over the cerebral hemispheres. The surface of the cerebral hemispheres is marked by ridges (*gyri*) and fissures (*sulci*) (see Fig. 5.5).

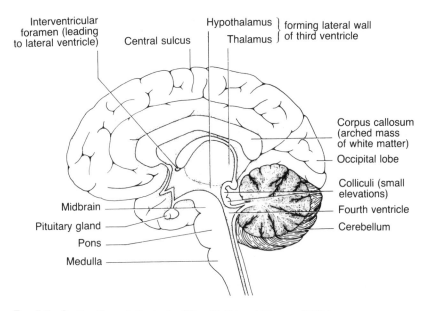

Fig. 5.5 Section through the brain. (After Moffat and Mottram 1987.)

It is composed of grey and white matter.

The *brainstem* connects the cerebral hemispheres with the spinal cord and consists of the:

- midbrain   the centre for visual reflexes.
- pons Varolii   a bridge of nerve matter.
- medulla oblongata   controling vital reflexes such as breathing, heart action, swallowing and vomiting.
- thalamus   where pain is felt.
- hypothalamus   an endocrine gland near the pituitary gland which controls the body rhythms.

The *cerebellum* or lesser brain, functions to co-ordinated muscular movement and balance. It is attached to the back of the brainstem and connected to the motor area of the cortex by way of the midbrain.

Meninges

This is the membrane that covers the brain and spinal cord. The meninges has three layers. These are the:

- pia mater   the inner layer.
- arachnoid   lying in the subarachnoid space or theca.
- dura mater   tough outer layer forming the venous sinuses and partitions known as falx cerebri and tentorium cerebri which give support and protection to the brain.

Cavities in the brain are known as *ventricles* and are filled with *cerebrospinal fluid* (csf).

The *choroid plexuses* are a network of minute capillary blood vessels which project into the ventricles and secrete cerebrospinal fluid.

Spinal cord

The spinal cord is about 18 inches (46 cm) long and 3/4 inch (2 cm) thick and serves the *spinal nerves*.

Nerve fibres passing from the lumbar and sacral regions form a cluster of fibres before they exit from the spinal canal resembling a horse's tail known as the *cauda equina*.

Like the brain the spinal cord is composed of grey and white matter.

Cranial nerves

There are 12 pairs of cranial nerves which include those of smell, sight and hearing. Some are motor nerves (i.e. resulting in initiating movement), some sensory (i.e. resulting in initiating the receipt of information from the senses) and some a mixture of both.

Spinal nerves

There are 31 pairs of spinal nerves. A pair of these nerves corresponds with each segment of the vertebral column.

The central nervous system is very complex with nerves supplying voluntary reflex action and also the involuntary nervous system dealing with the workings of the internal organs.

Arteries

The arteries of the skull named are:

basilar
cerebral
carotid
facial
temporal
occipital.

The arterial circle, also called the *circle of Willis*, is formed by branches of the cerebral arteries. It is located at the base of the brain.

The cardiovascular system

The cardiovascular system (CVS) comprises the:

* heart
* blood vessels.

Heart

A person's heart is about the size of their closed fist. It lies in the chest between the lungs with the bottom tip (apex) inclined to the left (see Fig. 5.6).

The heart is divided by a 'septum' into two sides, the right heart and the left heart. There should be no communication between the two sides after birth. Each side of the heart is further subdivided into two chambers, the upper is the *atrium* and the lower the *ventricle*.

The atrium and ventricle communicate by means of atrioventricular openings guarded by valves. On the right is the *tricuspid valve* and on the left the *mitral valve*.

The heart is surrounded by a membrane called the *pericardium*. The *myocardium* is the middle muscular layer and the *endocardium* the inner layer.

The interior of the ventricular walls have thickened columns of muscles (papillary muscles) and these are attached by thin tendinous cords (chordae tendineae) to the lower borders of the tricuspid and mitral valves.

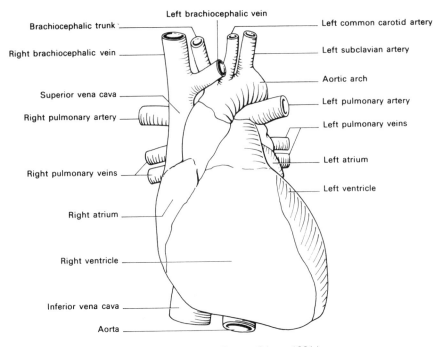

Fig. 5.6 The heart from the front. (*Source* Gibson 1981.)

Blood vessels

These are any 'tubes' carrying blood and the two major types are the:

● arteries
● veins.

The arteries carry oxygenated blood away from the heart to the organs and tissues of the body. Blood flows through the arteries which become increasingly smaller (arterioles) until a network of extremely fine capillaries is reached and the blood is then returned to the heart via venules (the very small veins) and veins. This is known as systemic circulation.

Pulmonary circulation concerns the circulation of blood between the heart and lungs via the pulmonary arteries and pulmonary veins. Here is the only case of where a vein carries oxygenated blood. In the lungs blood takes up oxygen from air breathed in and gives up carbon dioxide to be breathed out. The pulmonary arteries carry the blood (returning from the body) from the heart to the lungs. The oxygenated blood from the lungs is returned to the heart via the pulmonary veins to be pumped around the body.

Blood vessels attached to the heart are given below:

● The superior and inferior *venae cavae* empty their blood into the *right atrium*.

- The *pulmonary artery* carries blood away from the *right ventricle*.
- Four *pulmonary veins* bring blood from the lungs to the left atrium.
- The *aorta* carries blood away from the *left ventricle*.
- The openings of the aorta and pulmonary artery are guarded by *semi-lunar valves*.
- Blood supply to the heart is from the *coronary arteries*.
- Nerve supply is from the *vagus* and the *sympathetic nerves*.

Blood pressure

Blood pressure is the pressure exerted by blood within a blood vessel. It is influenced by the force with which the heart beats (the cardiac output) and the resistance to the flow of blood created by the blood vessels themselves.

It is measured in millimetres of mercury (mmHg) and has two elements, the systolic pressure and the diastolic pressure (see 'The cardiac cycle' below).

Cardiac cycle

The cardiac cycle is divided into two parts: contraction (systole) and relaxation (diastole).

- Two sounds may be heard during the action of the heart, the *systolic* sound and the *diastolic* sound.
- The cardiac impulse or apex beat starts at the sinoatrial (SA) node – a collection of highly specialized nerve tissue.
- The sinoatrial node often referred to as the 'pace-maker' of the heart.
- After passing the *atrioventricular* node this impulse passes to a special bundle of nerve and muscle fibres known as the *bundle of His*.
- In a condition known as heart block, the bundle of His fails to transmit the impulses so only one or two reach the arteries resulting in a very slow pulse.

Blood

Blood is pumped by the heart through all the arteries, veins, and capillaries. It carries oxygen, nutrients and hormones to the body's cells, and also removes the waste products.

Blood consists of:

- plasma
- blood cells.

Plasma

This is the clear, yellow fluid portion of the blood, free of cells. It represents 50% of the total blood volume and contains many essentials:

amino acids
glucose
protein
hormones
vitamins
minerals
urea and waste products
fibrinogen – a clotting factor.

Blood cells

These are:

- red cells (or erythrocytes)
- white cells (or leucocytes)
- platelets (or thrombocytes).

Red cells

These function primarily to carry oxygen around the body. They live for about 110 days, and originate in the bone marrow. The oxygen is carried as part of an iron-containing compound, haemoglobin.

White cells

These cells are part of the body's defence system, destroying bacteria, viruses and toxins, and activating the body's immune responses. There are five types of cell, classified according to the presence (or not) of granules:

granulocytes   neutrophils, basophils, eosinophils
agranulocytes   monocytes, lymphocytes.

The lymphocytes are active members of the body's immune system. There are two distinct types of lymphocytes: B-cells and T-cells. The B-cells search out, identify and 'hand-cuff' themselves to specific antibody-producing bodies (known as 'antigens'). T-cells assist B-cells and are sometimes called 'killer' cells because they secrete immunologically essential chemicals.

Lymphocytes normally account for 25% of the total white cell count, but increase in numbers in response to infection.

Platelets

These cells are essential for blood clotting.

Blood serum

If a sample of blood is left standing undisturbed, the cells will soon coagulate and collect at the bottom, leaving a thick sticky fluid above. This is the blood serum.

Blood groups

There are many blood grouping systems, but the most clinically important is the ABO grouping system. There are blood types A, B, AB, and O (with many subdivisions), determined by the presence or absence of two-antibody-forming proteins ('antigens'), A and B. Group A has antigen A, group B, has B, group AB has both, and group O has neither antigens.

The presence or absence of these antibody-triggering chemicals in the blood (in other words, someone's blood group) becomes important when a blood transfusion is – or might be (e.g. during surgery) – necessary. If someone is given blood that is not of the same group as his, then a severe antibody reaction can set in as the person's body tries to attack the alien blood. This is a very serious condition and can lead to death.

Blood is also either rhesus positive (Rh pos) or rhesus negative (Rh neg). Most of the population in the UK is rhesus positive – which means that the rhesus factor is present in their blood. Rhesus-negative people may develop

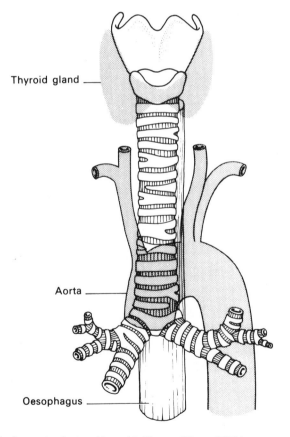

Fig. 5.7 The larynx, trachea and bronchi. (*Source* Gibson 1981.)

antibodies in their blood during pregnancies (i.e. if the baby is rhesus positive) or after blood transfusions with rhesus-positive blood. The subject is very complex, but these antibodies can be dealt with much more successfully today than previously.

The respiratory system

The respiratory system (RS), see Fig. 5.7, consists of:

- nose
- nasopharynx
- larynx
- trachea
- bronchi
- lungs.

(See also the ear, nose and throat section at the end of this chapter.)

Nose

The nostrils (anterior nares) form the external entrance and lead into two nasal cavities separated by a septum. The turbinate bones (nasal conchae) project into the nasal cavity.

Nasopharynx

The nasopharynx is part of the pharynx lying behind the nose and communicates with the nasal cavity.

Larynx

The larynx (voice box) is composed of thyroid cartilage, epiglottis, cricoid cartilage and two arytenoid cartilages. It is situated at the top of the trachea, below the root of the tongue and hyoid bone (small bone in the neck).

Trachea

The trachea (windpipe) is an air passage about 10 cm long extending from the throat and larynx to the main bronchi.

Bronchi

The bronchi (single bronchus) are any of the larger passages containing air to and within the lungs.

Lungs

The two lungs are the principal organs of respiration. It is here that a process called gaseous exchange takes place. Moist, warm oxygen-rich air enters the lungs and via the alveoli the blood stream to reach the cells, and waste carbon dioxide is excreted out of the body via the lungs.

The lungs lie in the thoracic cavity. The *mediastinum* is the space between the lungs in the thoracic cavity and contains the heart. The *diaphragm* lies between the thoracic and abdominal cavities and is the chief muscle of inspiration. The lobes of the lung consist of ramifications and terminations of the bronchi, *alveoli* (air sacs), blood vessels, lymphatic and areolar tissue. The *pleura* surrounds each lung. It is a double membrane and between the two layers there is a slight exudate which lubricates the surface preventing friction between the lungs and the chest wall during breathing. Normally the two layers of pleura are in contact with each other but in some lung conditions there may be fluid or air between the two layers (pneumothorax).

The gastrointestinal system

The gastrointestinal (GI) system consists of the:

- oesophagus ⎫
- stomach ⎬ gastrointestinal tract
- small intestine ⎪
- large intestine ⎭
- liver
- gall bladder
- pancreas.

Oesophagus

The oesophagus is a muscular tube about 25 cm long. Food passes along the mouth, through the oropharynx and laryngeal pharynx to reach the oesophagus, where it is then propelled along to the stomach.

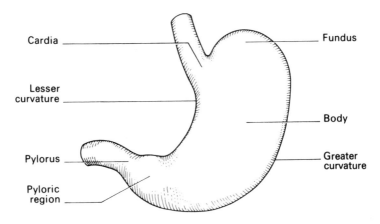

Fig. 5.8 The stomach. (*Source* Gibson 1981.)

Stomach

The stomach (see Fig. 5.8) communicates at the inlet with the oesophagus by means of a purse-string-like sphincter, the *cardiac sphincter* and at the outlet with the duodenum by the *pyloric sphincter*. The stomach consists of two parts: the *fundus* and the pyloric *antrum*.

The stomach lies below the diaphragm, in front of the pancreas, and the spleen lies against the left side of the fundus.

The stomach wall is thickly lined with *rugae mucosa* to protect it from its own very acid digestive juices. It is in the stomach that food is broken down for its nutrient parts to be absorbed and used by the body.

Small intestine

The small intestine is a tube about 6 m (20 ft) long. It extends from the stomach to the ileocaecal valve where it joins the large intestine.

It is divided into three important parts; the:

duodenum
jejunum
ileum.

The *duodenum* is the first part lying below the pylorus.

The *jejunum* occupies the next section and the *ileum* is in the final section joining the large intestine at the ileocaecal valve.

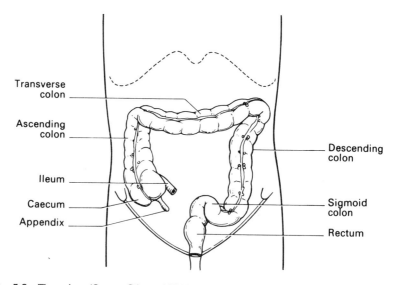

Fig. 5.9   The colon. (*Source* Gibson 1981.)

Large intestine (colon)

The *caecum* is the beginning of the large intestine to which the vestigial appendix is attached (see Fig. 5.9).

The caecum lies in the right iliac region and the pain and tenderness in appendicitis is normally felt in the right iliac fossa (RIF).

The *ascending colon* turns at the hepatic flexure into the *transverse colon*. The transverse colon turns at the splenic flexure into the *descending colon*. In the left iliac region a bend called the sigmoid flexure or *sigmoid colon* is formed. It then enters the true pelvis and becomes the *rectum*. The rectum is the lowest 12 cm of the large intestine and ends at the *anal canal*. The opening, the *anus* is guarded by sphincter muscles.

Peritoneum

The *peritoneum* is a double membrane which lines the walls of the abdominal cavity and pelvis.

The *omenta* are three double folds of peritoneum which separate some organs from each other.

The *mesenteries* are folds of peritoneum which join the different parts of the intestines and act as a support. They contain numerous lymphatic glands and mesenteric blood vessels.

Liver

The liver is the largest gland in the body and is divided into two main lobes, right and left. It is situated in the abdominal cavity on the right beneath the diaphragm. It has several important functions including the modification and storage of food material, detoxication of harmful substances and the production and destruction of red blood cells.

Gall bladder

The gall bladder is a pear-shaped organ on the under surface of the liver. It acts as a reservoir for bile. A duct leading from the gall bladder joins the hepatic duct and forms the common bile duct which conveys bile to the duodenum.

Pancreas

The pancreas is vital to life and has two important functions, the secretion of an important digestive fluid and the manufacture of hormones, such as insulin.

The endocrine system

The major *endocrine glands* are the:

- hypothalamus
- pituitary
- gonads (testes in the male; ovaries in the female)
- thyroid
- parathyroid
- pancreas (part of).

Endocrine glands are ductless organs which release their secretions (hormones) directly into the circulatory system. These hormones are very important in controlling metabolism and other body processes.

Hypothalamus

The hypothalamus lies near the pituitary deep in the brain and directs the body's many rhythms.

Pituitary gland

Also, deep in the brain, the pituitary gland rests on the sella turcica, a depression in the sphenoid bone. The anterior lobe secretes hormones related to growth and the function of the other endocrine glands. The posterior lobe of the pituitary secretes two hormones, oxytocin and vasopressin (or antidiuretic hormone). The pituitary is also called the hypophysis.

Reproductive glands (gonads)

The testes and ovaries, are controlled by the gonadotrophic hormone of the pituitary and secrete testosterone in the male and oestrogen and progesterone in the female.

Thyroid gland

The thyroid consists of two lobes on each side of the trachea connected by a strip of tissue called the isthmus. Deficiency or overproduction of its secretion thyroxine can cause serious metabolic disorders – namely, myxoedema and thyrotoxicosis.

Parathyroid glands

These are four small glands, two each side of the thyroid. They regulate the amount of calcium in blood and bone via the production of parathyroid hormone.

Adrenal glands

These sit on top of each kidney. They produce the hormones cortisol and adrenaline.

Pancreas

As well as having an important role in the digestive system, the pancreas contains the Islets of Langerhans which secrete insulin. Lack of insulin causes a form of diabetes mellitus.

Pineal gland or body

Again, located deep within the brain, the pineal gland is now thought to be an endocrine gland. Its function, however, remains obscure.

Thymus

This is a ductless gland-like body lying beneath the breastbone and has a role in the immune system of the body.

The genitourinary system

The genitourinary system comprises the urinary system and the reproductive system.

The urinary system

The urinary system deals with the collection, retention and expulsion of waste fluid from the body – urine. It consists of the:

- kidneys
- ureters
- bladder
- urethra.

Kidneys

The kidneys are a pair of bean-shaped organs lying in the rear (posterior) part of the abdomen on either side of the spinal column. In most people, the left kidney is slightly higher than the right because of the presence of the liver on the right side. There is an outer cortical part and an inner medullary part which contains the nephrons.

The kidney's function is to produce and eliminate urine by means of a complex filtration and reabsorption system. More than 1000 litres of blood pass through the kidneys every day. Water is removed as urine and filtered water returned to the blood. The kidneys thus play an important part in the balance of water in the body.

The kidneys also manufacture a substance (erythropoietin) necessary for the formation of red blood cells.

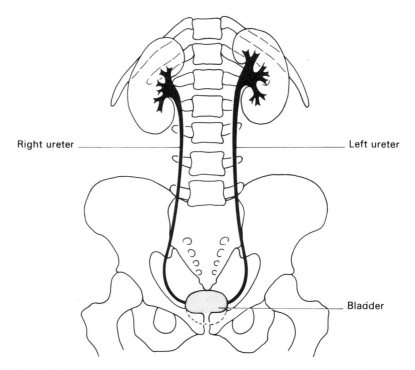

Fig. 5.10   The ureters as shown by intravenous pyelogram. (*Source* Gibson 1981.)

Ureters

These are the pair of tubes that convey the urine from the kidneys to the bladder (see Fig. 5.10).

Bladder

The bladder is a muscular sac which acts as a reservoir for urine until the bladder is emptied. The expulsion of urine (micturition) is normally under conscious voluntary control, and is a complex co-ordinated process. Special stretch sensors tell the person (via the spinal cord and brain) when the bladder is due for emptying.

Urethra

This is the external urinary opening, or meatus, connecting the bladder to the outside and through which the urine flows during micturition.

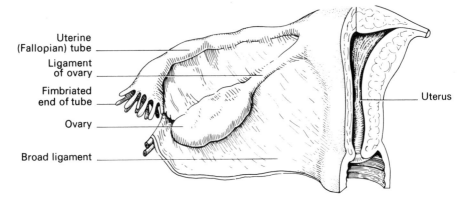

Fig. 5.11　The female reproductive organs within the pelvis. (*Source* Gibson 1981.)

The reproductive system

Female

The female reproductive system (see Fig. 5.11) may be divided into:

- external organs
- internal organs.

The external organs
The external organs are collectively known as the vulva and comprise the:

- mons pubis
- labia majora
- labia minora
- clitoris
- perineum.

The *mons pubis* (mons veneris) is the pad of fat lying in front of the pubic bone (symphysis pubis). It becomes covered with hair at puberty.

The *labia majora* are the two fleshy lips forming the side of the vulva. Two glands, *Bartholin's glands*, lie on each side towards the back. These become active with sexual arousal and lubricate the entrance to the vagina.

Labia minora are the two more delicate folds between the upper parts of the labia majora. The *fourchette* is a small fold joining them near the anus.

The *clitoris* is the small highly sensitive body tucked at the front of the vulva between the labia minora. It is made of erectile tissue, like the penis in the male, but unlike the penis has a sexual function only.

The *perineum* is the area between the vagina and the rectum.

The *hymen* is a thin fold of mucous membrane, skin and fibrous tissue at the vaginal introitus (entrance).

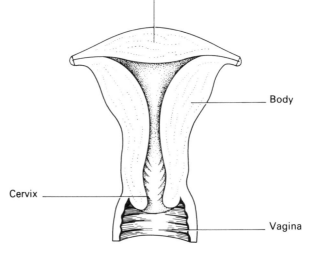

Fundus of uterus

Body

Cervix

Vagina

Fig. 5.12   Section through the uterus. (*Source* Gibson 1981.)

The internal organs
The internal organs comprise the:

- vagina
- uterus
- fallopian tubes
- ovaries.

The *vagina* is a muscular, ribbed tube extending between the introitus at the vulva and the uterus. It is rather like an empty sleeve but will balloon and extend with arousal to accommodate an erect penis. It is also the birth canal and will stretch to allow the passage of a baby at birth. It surrounds the lower part of the cervix. Small recesses in front and at the side of the cervix are called *fornices*.

In front (anterior) of the vagina is the urethra and base of the bladder. Behind (posterior) is the rectum and *pouch of Douglas*.

The vagina protects itself from ill health by its slightly acid environment (pH) and its special indigenous bacteria.

The *uterus* (Fig. 5.12) is a pear-shaped organ made up of an intricate lattice of muscles. It is supported by ligaments and 'sits' in a hammock of muscles on the floor of the pelvis ('pelvic floor'). The uterus consists of a:

cervix
body
fundus.

The cervix is continuous with the body of the uterus above by the *internal os* and below with the vagina by the *external os*.

The uterus is lined with a mucous membrane called the *endometrium*. It is the endometrium that is shed every month at menstruation or proliferates to support and nourish the 'nesting' fertilized egg or embryo should pregnancy occur.

The *Fallopian tubes* are about 20 cm long and are narrow at the uterine end. They then enlarge forming an ampulla and finally bend downwards to end in a fringed (fimbriated) margin. One of the 'fringes' (fimbriae) is attached to the ovary. The fallopian tubes propel the released egg along towards the uterus. Infection in the fallopian tubes is known as salpingitis.

The *ovaries* are two almond-shaped glands on each side of the uterus, below the fallopian tubes. They are composed of Graafian follicles embedded in a stroma. Maturation of the Graafian follicle and liberation of the ovum is termed ovulation. Oophoritis is inflammation of the ovary. The ovaries also produce the female hormones oestrogen and progesterone.

The term *adnexa* refers to the uterine appendages, ovaries, tubes and ligaments. 'No adnexal masses' is quite frequently used in gynaecological reports.

Male

The external organs
The external organs consist of the:

- penis
- scrotum
- testes.

The *penis* contains the urinary urethra, passing through the prostate gland on its way to the external opening (meatus). The penis also contains many blood vessels and erectile tissue for its function as the organ of insemination.

The loose skin covering the penis is the *prepuce* or *foreskin*. Infection of this is known as balanitis. Phimosis is a tightening of the foreskin so that it cannot be pulled back. Circumcision is the surgical removal of the foreskin.

The *scrotum* is the pouch situated behind the penis which houses the testes. Held away from the body the testes are kept at a lower temperature which is conducive to sperm production (see Fig. 5.13).

The *testes* (singular = testis) are male organs of reproduction in which spermatozoa are formed and male sex hormones are produced. Orchitis is inflammation of the testis.

The internal organs
The internal organs consist of the:

- seminal vesicles
- epididymis
- vans deferens
- prostate gland.

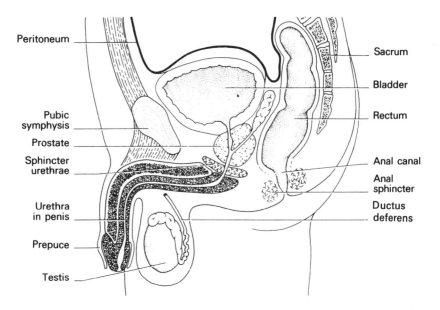

Fig. 5.13   The male reproductive and genitourinary organs. (*Source* Moffat and Mottram 1987.)

The *seminal vesicles* serve as a reservoir for the secretions of the testes.

The *epididymis* is a small collecting organ lying near the testes and attached to it.

The *vas deferens* is the tube passing from the epididymis to the seminal vesicle. It is cut at a vasectomy operation.

The *prostate gland* lies below the bladder surrounding the urethra. The glands of the prostate secrete a fluid which mingles with the secretion of the testes.

The lymphatic system

The purpose of the lymphatic system is to drain tissue spaces and absorb fat. It also defends the body against infection.

Lymph

As the blood circulates a considerable amount of blood fluid exudes through the walls of minute capillaries to bathe the tissues. This is called *lymph* and it is collected and carried back to the blood stream by the lymphatic system.

Lymph vessels and nodes

Lymphatic vessels are rather similar to small veins. Lymphatic glands (nodes) are placed in the course of the vessels and contain reticuloendothelial cells.

The main lymph nodes lie in the neck, axilla, thorax, abdomen and groin. They can become swollen and inflamed in the presence of infection.

Spleen

As the spleen contains mainly lymphatic tissue it is included here. The spleen is situated in the upper part of the abdomen on the left side. It performs various tasks including the disintegration of old red blood cells (setting free the haemoglobin – protein in the blood which contains a pigment rich in iron), blood storage, the manufacture of white blood cells and immune system blood cells.

The reticuloendothelial system

This is a diffuse collection of cells occurring throughout the body and includes the lymphocytes and phagocytic cells. They are the first line of defence against foreign particles and bacteria. They also destroy worn out blood cells. Reticuloendothelial cells may be found in:

blood vessel walls
bone marrow
liver
lymph nodes
spleen
thymus.

Most of these organs/tissues have been dealt with elsewhere but bone marrow is mentioned here for completeness. *Bone marrow* is a soft filling of bones. Red bone marrow manufacturers red blood cells and infection fighting cells. A bone marrow transplant involves the removal of healthy marrow from a donor and infusion intravenously into the patient.

The ear, nose and throat system

The ear, nose and throat (ENT) system is dealt with only briefly here. The paranasal sinuses are the only part of the 'nose' considered here. For more details about the nasal passage the reader is referred to the earlier section on 'The respiratory system'.

Nose

See 'The respiratory system' dealt with earlier in this chapter.

Ears

The ear is the organ of hearing and the nerve supplying this sense is the auditory or eighth cranial nerve (see Fig. 5.14). The ear is divided into three parts:

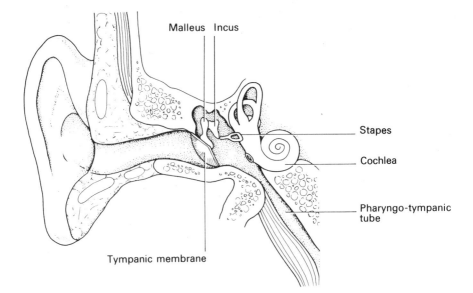

Fig. 5.14 The ear. (*Source* Gibson 1981.)

external ear
middle ear
internal ear

External ear
The external ear consists of the auricle or pinna which is the projecting part on the outside of the head, and the external auditory or acoustic meatus.

Middle ear
The middle ear or tympanic cavity is a chamber internal to the tympanic membrane or eardrum, and contains air. It communicates with the mastoid antrum, and by two Eustachian or pharyngotympanic tubes, one on each side, with the pharynx. The openings of these tubes are normally closed but open on swallowing. In this way the pressure in the middle ear is kept the same as the atmospheric pressure. The middle ear communicates with the internal or inner ear by the oval window (fenestra ovalis) and the round window (fenestra rotunda).

The auditory ossicles are three small bones across the middle ear called the malleus (hammer), incus (anvil) and stapes (stirrup), so called because of their resemblance to these objects.

Inner ear
The internal ear is the organ of hearing and consists of several cavities called osseous or bony labyrinth lined by membranes, (membranous labyrinth).

In the labyrinth or inner ear is the cochlea, a spiral tube resembling the shell of a snail which contains the nerves that transmit sound to the brain. Also contained within the inner ear are the semicircular canals and the movement of fluid in these canals affects balance.

The organ of Corti receives the nerve endings of the auditory nerve which is divided into two parts, the vestibular nerve concerned with balance and the cochlear nerve, the true nerve of hearing, known together as the vestibulocochlear (8th cranial) nerve.

Paranasal sinuses

The paranasal sinuses consist of four pairs, maxillary, frontal, sphenoid and ethmoid, situated in the cranial bones of these names.

Throat

The throat consists of the fauces, passage from mouth to pharynx, pharynx and larynx. The palatine tonsils (normally referred to as tonsils) are partially imbedded in the mucous membrane at the back of the throat. At the back of the tongue are the lingual tonsils and on the upper rear wall of the mouth cavity are the adenoids (pharyngeal tonsils).

The eye

The eye (see Fig. 5.15) is the organ of sight and the optic or second cranial nerve is the sensory nerve of sight.

The eyeball is contained within the bony orbit and protected by append-ages such as eyelids, eyebrows, conjunctiva and lachrimal apparatus. The eye is moved by six muscles, superior, inferior, internal and external rectus muscles, and superior oblique and inferior oblique muscles.

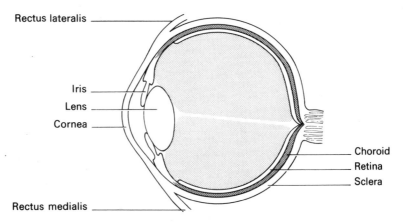

Fig. 5.15 The eye. (*Source* Gibson 1981.)

The eyeball has three coverings:

- sclera   tough outer fibrous coat forming the white of the eye.
- choroid   middle coat containing blood vessels and the pigment which gives colour to the eye. Just behind the iris it is thickened to form the ciliary body.
- retina   the inner coat composed of layers of nerve fibres, nerve cells, rods and cones. A yellow spot called the macula is the part of the retina that is responsible for accurate central vision.

In examining the eye from front to back the following parts are seen, the:

- cornea   transparent front portion continuous with the dense white sclera.
- anterior chamber   between cornea the iris.
- iris   coloured curtain in front of the lens continuous with the choroid coat.
- pupil   dark central spot which is an opening in the iris through which light reaches the retina.
- posterior chamber   between iris and lens.
- aqueous humour   this fluid is derived from the ciliary body and a tiny vein called canal of Schlemm takes the fluid back to be re-absorbed in the blood stream.
- lens   a biconvex transparent body of several layers behind the iris.
- vitreous humour   remaining back portion of the eyeball filled with jelly-like fluid.

Appendages

- *Eyebrows*   the eyebrows are attached to muscles beneath and help to protect the eye from too much light, foreign objects and perspiration.
- *Eyelids*   two tarsal plates form the eyelids which are covered by skin and lined by conjunctiva. Eyelashes are attached to the margins of the lids. Two muscles move the eyelids, the levator palpebrae and the orbicularis palpebrae.
- *Conjunctiva*   this is a mucous membrane lining the eyelids.
- *Lachrimal apparatus*   lachrimal glands secrete the tears. As the eyelids move in blinking, the tears are distributed across the surface of the eyeball. Excess fluid passes into the lachrymal duct and then by the nasolachrymal duct into the nose.

Chapter 6
Medical Terminology: Key Word Elements

It is important to become thoroughly familiar with the following root words, prefixes and suffixes. The meaning and spelling of many medical words will then become clear.

At the end of this chapter there is a list of words not previously shown in the examples. Once you have studied this section, you should be able to understand their meaning without further explanation.

Meanings of medical prefixes with examples

Prefix	Meaning	Example	Meaning
aden-	gland	adenopathy	enlargement of the glands, usually lymph glands
adip-	fat	adipose	fatty
angi-	vessel	angiogram	X-ray of blood vessels
ante-	before	ante-natal	before birth
arthr-	joint	arthritis	inflammation of the joint
bi-	twice	bilateral	both sides
blephar-	eyelid	blepharitis	inflammation of the eyelids
brady-	slow	bradycardia	slow heart beat, slow pulse
bronch-	windpipe	bronchitis	infection of one or more bronchi
bucc-	cheek	buccal	pertaining to the cheek
carcin-	cancer	carcinoma	malignant new growth (often written Ca.)
cardi-	heart	cardiac	pertaining to the heart
cephal-	head	cephalic	pertaining to the head
cer-	wax	cerumen	wax-like secretion found in the ear
cerebr-	brain	cerebral	pertaining to the brain
chol-	bile	cholecystitis	inflammation of the gall bladder which stores bile
chondr-	cartilage	chondritis	inflammation of a cartilage
colp-	hollow	colposcopy	looking into the vagina and cervix with a colposcope
cost-	rib	costal	pertaining to a rib or ribs
crani-	skull	cranial	pertaining to the skull

Prefix	Meaning	Example	Meaning
cyan-	blue	cyanosis	blue discoloration due to lack of oxygen
cyst-	a bladder	cystoscopy	examining the bladder with a cystoscope
dactyl-	finger or toe	dactylomegaly	abnormally large fingers or toes
dent-	tooth	dental	pertaining to a tooth or teeth
derm-	skin	dermatology	medical speciality concerned with treatment of the skin
dys-	painful, difficult	dysmenorrhoea	painful periods
endo-	inside	endometrium	inner lining of the uterus
febr-	fever	febrile	feverish
ferr-	iron	ferritin	chief form in which iron is stored in the body
galact-	milk	galactorrhoea	excessive flow of milk from the breast
gastr-	stomach	gastrectomy	removal of the stomach
gloss-	tongue	glossal	pertaining to the tongue
gnath-	jaw	gnathic	pertaining to the jaw
haem-	relating to blood	haemoglobin	oxygen carrying pigment of red blood cell
hepat-	liver	hepatitis	inflammation of the liver
hydro-	relating to water	hydramnios	excess amniotic fluid around fetus
hyper-	above	hypertension	high blood pressure
hypno-	sleep	hypnotic	inducing sleep (e.g. hypnotic drug)
hypo-	below	hypothyroid	deficient of thyroid activity
hyster-	womb	hysterectomy	removal of the uterus
inter-	between	intervertebral	between the vertebra
intra-	within	intravenous	injection into a vein
labi-	lip	labial	pertaining to a lip (commonly the labia of the vulva)
leuco-	white	leucocytes	white blood cells
lingu-	tongue	lingual	referring to the tongue
litho	stone	lithotripsy	crushing of a stone
macro-	large	macroscopy	examining with the naked eye not microscope
mal-	bad	malfunction	failure to function in the right way
mamm-	breast	mammogram	X-ray of breasts
mast-	breast	mastectomy	removal of a breast
melan-	black	melanoma	dark mole-like tumour
mes-	middle	mesial	to the middle
micro-	small	microscopic	too small to be visible to the naked eye
my-	muscle	myalgia	pain in a muscle or muscles
myco-	fungoid	mycosis	any disease caused by a fungus
myel-	marrow	myeloblast	cell found in bone marrow
nephr-	kidney	nephrectomy	removal of a kidney

Prefix	Meaning	Example	Meaning
neuro-	nerve	neuroma	tumour of nerve cells and fibres
olig-	little	oligospermia	scanty spermatozoa
oo-	egg	oophorectomy	removal of an ovary
orchi-	testicle	orchidectomy	removal of a testicle
oss/ost-	relating to bone	osseous	bony
oto-	relating to the ear	otology	branch of medicine dealing with the ear
par-	bear	parous	having borne one or more viable children
per-	through	per mouth	taken orally
peri	around	periorbital	situated around the orbit or eye socket
phleb-	vein	phlebitis	inflammation of a vein
pneumo-	air	pneumothorax	accummulation of air in the pleural space
poly-	much	polyuria	passage of large volumes of urine
presby-	old	presbycusis	loss of hearing due to old age
proct-	anus	proctoscope	instrument inserted through anus to visually examine rectum
psych-	mind/soul	psychiatry	study and treatment of mental illness
pto-	fall	ptosis	drooping of the upper eyelid
py-	pus	pyemia	septicaemia with multiple abscesses
retro-	backwards	retroverted	turned backwards
rhin-	nose	rhinitis	inflammation of the mucous membrane of the nose
salping	tube	salpingitis	infection of Fallopian tube
scler-	hard	scleroderma	hardening of connective tissues of many organs
somat-	body	somatic	pertaining to the body
splen-	spleen	splenectomy	removal of the spleen
sten-	narrow	stenosis	narrowing
stom-	mouth	stomatitis	inflammation of the mouth
sub-	under	subcostal	under the ribs
super-	above	supernumerary	in excess of the normal number
thorac-	chest	thoracic	pertaining to the chest (thorax)
thromb-	lump/clot	thrombosis	formation of a clot of blood (thrombus)
trich-	hair	trichosis	any disease or abnormal growth of hair
vesic-	bladder	vesical	pertaining to the bladder

Meanings of medical suffixes with examples

Suffix	Meaning	Example	Meaning
-algia	relating to pain	neuralgia	nerve pain usually in head or face
-cele/ -coele	hernia of	meningocele	hernial protrusion of the meninges
-centesis	puncture	amniocentesis	puncture of the amnion to obtain amniotic fluid
-cyte	relating to a cell	leucocyte	white blood cell
-dynia	having pain	coccydynia	painful condition of coccyx
-ectomy	removal of	appendicectomy	removal of appendix
-itis	inflammation of	cystitis	inflammation of the bladder
-malacia	softening	osteomalacia	softening of the bones
-megaly	large	cardiomegaly	enlarged heart
-oma	tumour	adenoma	tumour composed of glandular tissue
-opia	relating to vision	myopia	short sight
-opsia	sight	achromatopsia	colour blindness
-oscopy	looking into	colonoscopy	looking into the colon
-ostomy	making an opening	colostomy	opening in colon to surface of body
-otomy	cutting into	vagotomy	cutting into the vagus nerve
-pathy	disease of	lymphadenopathy	swelling of lymph gland
-pexy	fixing	orchidopexy	fixing an undescended testicle in the scrotum
-plasty	repair of	arthroplasty	repair of a joint
-plegia	paralysis	paraplegia	paralysis of the lower part of the body
-rrhaphy	sewing up	herniorrhaphy	repair of a hernia
-rrhage	excessive flow	haemorrhage	excessive bleeding
-rrhoea	flowing	diarrhoea	fluid stools
-uria	relating to urine	haematuria	blood in the urine

List of words whose meanings should now be clear

arthralgia
bronchoscopy
chondromalacia
colporrhaphy
cystocoele
dysuria
gastrostomy
hepatomegaly
hydrocephalic
mastopexy

micropsia
myopathy
nephroma
oliguria
otorrhoea
presbyopia
proctitis
salpingo-oophorectomy
thorocotomy

Chapter 7
Medical Investigations Used in Diagnosis

In order to arrive at a correct diagnosis of the patient's symptoms and to make certain no serious underlying cause has been missed, it is often necessary to carry out a large number of investigations. Many of these investigations are blood tests and it is helpful to the secretary in the audio-typing of letters and reports, to be familiar with many of them. The secretary should also know the department to contact if asked to obtain a result of a particular test.

Chemical Pathology (Biochemistry)

Investigations concerned with the chemistry of the body are performed by the Chemical Pathology Laboratory (Biochemistry). Some of the following blood chemistry tests may be ordered:

amylase
aspartate aminotransferase (AST)
bicarbonate
bilirubin
calcium
cardiac enzymes (creatinine kinase (CK) lactate dehydrogenase (LD))
chloride
cholesterol
creatinine
follicle stimulating hormone
fructosamine
glucose
gamma(γ-)GT
iron (ferritin)
luteinizing hormone
magnesium
phosphatase (acid or alkaline)
phosphate
potassium
prolactin
proteins (total and albumin)
protein bound iodine (PBI)
T_4 (serum thyroxine)

TSH – thyroid stimulating hormone
transaminases (glutamic-oxaloacetic (GOT) and glutamic-pyruvic (GPT))
testosterone
triglyceride
urate
urea

The levels of oxygen and carbon dioxide in a patient's blood (blood gases) may be measured in the biochemistry laboratory, from a sample of arterial blood (blood taken from an artery).

Urine may be examined to determine the levels of calcium, creatinine, protein and steroids.

Faeces are analyzed for fat content.

Cerebrospinal fluid (csf) may be examined for protein and glucose.

The absence or presence and amount of many 'chemicals' in the body can be indicative of disease or give important clues as to what may be wrong with a patient.

Examples of many of these tests will be found in the medical summaries in Chapter 10.

Common abbreviations

Terms connected with biochemical investigations which are useful to know include:

U & Es   urea and electrolytes. Electrolytes in the body fluids are sodium, potassium, calcium, magnesium, chloride, bicarbonate and phosphate.

Electrophoresis is a common investigative technique.

GTT   glucose tolerance test.

LFTs   liver function tests.

Symbols used in biochemistry results

mmol	millimole
mmol/l	millimole per litre
nmol	nanamole
µmol	micromole
U or IU	international unit
>	more than
<	less than

Haematology

The Haematology Department performs tests concerned with blood cells (see Chapter 5). Most blood tests are performed on venous blood (blood taken from a vein).

Blood counts

The main groups of blood cells are the:

erythrocytes   red, iron-rich blood cells
leucocytes   white, infection-fighting cells
platelets   clotting blood cells.

Erythrocytes

The iron compound in the blood that carries oxygen to the cells (and carbon dioxide away to the lungs) is called *haemoglobin*. The haemoglobin (Hb) content of red blood cells is assessed in a number of conditions. If it is below the agreed normal level the patient is regarded as anaemic of which there are many forms.

Normal Hb levels are:

Men   13.5–18.0 g/dl (grams per decilitre)
Women   11.5–16.0 g/dl

Leucocytes

The white blood cells play an important part in fighting infections by ingesting bacteria. When infection is present the white cell count is normally raised.

Platelets

The platelets (also sometimes called 'thrombocytes') are involved in the clotting mechanism of the blood.

Common abbreviations

When a doctor requests a full and differential blood count on a patient, the results will come back with figures attached to the following abbreviations:

FBC   Full blood count
ESR   Erythrocyte sedimentation rate
MCV   Mean corpuscular volume
RBC   Red blood count
WBC   White blood count.

Blood transfusions

The Haematology Department tests and matches ('cross-matching') blood for transfusions. (See also Chapter 5.)

A sample of the patient's blood will be sent to Haematology for cross-matching before surgery and any major procedure.

Blood diseases

Patients who attend the Haematology clinic regularly are usually suffering from blood diseases such as leukaemia, all forms of anaemia, disorders of the bone marrow or lymphoid tissue and those needing or being treated with anticlotting (anticoagulant) drugs. These patients will probably be on drugs such as heparin or warfarin to prevent clotting in cases of venous thrombosis or prosthetic heart valves.

Some black patients may suffer from sickle-cell anaemia; people from Mediterranean countries may have – or carry the gene for – a hereditary anaemia known as β-thalassaemia; tests for these conditions are frequently performed.

Patients suffering from pernicious anaemia have a deficiency of vitamin B_{12}; a deficiency in folates (folic acid) leads to another type of anaemia so these are further examples of tests carried out in Haematology.

Clinical measurements

Such tests include lung function tests expecially in those suffering from chronic obstructive airways disease (COAD); urine flow and urodynamic studies on patients with incontinence, urgency, frequency, hypotonic and unstable bladder.

Cytogenics

Chromosome studies are carried out in the Cytogenic Unit. Not all hospitals have such a unit and specimens have to be sent to the nearest laboratory by arrangement.

Normally there are 46 chromosomes in the cells of the body. XX or XY is described as a normal karyotype. X is the female sex chromosome and Y the male chromosome. The word *trisomy* denotes the presence of an additional cell which can cause many forms of abnormality. Trisomy-21 results in Down's syndrome.

Amniotic fluid (fluid around the fetus) is sent for chromosome studies in some patients around the 16–18th week of pregnancy. Chromosome abnormalities and the sex of the child can then be ascertained. The sex of the child may be important where there is a family history of an X- or Y-chromosome-linked disorder (e.g. sickle-cell trait; Hunter's syndrome).

Cytology

The Cytology Department examines cervical smears, body fluids, and sometimes blood, for malignant cells or cells showing precancerous change.

Electrocardiogram

Electrocardiograms (ECGs) are frequently ordered to detect abnormalities of the heart action in medical patients and often as a routine before surgery.

Electroencephalogram

Electroencephalogram (EEG) measurement of the brain waves may be ordered for patients suffering from epilepsy and other neurological disorders.

Gastroenterology/Endoscopy

Most hospitals have an Endoscopy Unit where patients undergo investigative procedures on a day-case basis.

Endoscopic (visual examination of any cavity of the body with an endoscope) examination of the oesophagus, stomach and duodenum is performed to detect inflammation, ulcers and tumours, and to take biopsies of suspicious tissue for histology.

Colonoscopy is likewise performed to take biopsies and to diagnose conditions of the colon such as ulcerative colitis. Crohn's disease, diverticulitis, polyps and tumours.

Endoscopes, colonoscopes and bronchoscopes are long flexible tubes that relay images via fibreoptics on to an eye piece or TV screen.

Sigmoidoscopy and proctoscopy (examinations of the large intestine and rectum) are usually carried out at an outpatient clinical examination.

Other endoscopies

Bronchoscopy is examination of the bronchi and lungs.

Colposcopy is examination of the vagina and cervix by means of a colposcope. Abnormal areas are then treated by laser. Colposcopy is normally performed in an outpatient operating session in the gynaecological department.

Cystoscopy is examination of the bladder.

Histology

The Histology Department performs microscopic examination on all tissue removed from the body – for example on tumours, organs, and curettings (scrapings).

Microbiology

The Micorobiology Laboratory is concerned with infection with microorganisms, such as bacteria and viruses. There may be additional laboratories specializing in bacteriology or virology.

Infectious diseases

Tests for all infectious diseases are carried out in this department, such as tests for hepatitis B, the AIDS virus (HIV) and sexually transmitted diseases including related diseases using RPR (rapid plasma reagin) – a screening test for syphilis – and TPHA (*Treponema pallidum* haemagglutination test) – a test for the causative organism of syphilis. Both RPR and TPHA tests are routinely carried out on antenatal patients when booking in at the hospital. Levels of antibodies (antibody titres) against infections such as rubella (German measles) are also determined.

Specimens

All specimens must be clearly labelled and the site and nature of the specimen also marked. Many specimens sent to Microbiology are swabs from wounds and from the nose, throat or vagina if infection is suspected. Swabs will always state where they have been taken from – e.g. HVS is a high vaginal swab. Sputum and other body fluids can also be examined for organisms – e.g. sputum for acid-fast bacilli (afb) an indication of tuberculosis.

Urine specimens may be a:

CSU   catheter specimen of urine
EMU   early morning urine
MSU   mid-stream specimen of urine.

This gives the microbiologist important information as to the likelihood of certain 'normal' bacteria being present.

Cerebrospinal fluid (csf) is examined for bacteria and viruses in cases of suspected meningitis.

Stool samples are sent for culture, for example, in suspected salmonella or other bowel infections.

Specimens likely to contain bacteria are usually sent for 'M C & S' – microscopy, culture and sensitivity. The subsequent report will identify the organism and list the drugs to which it is sensitive and resistant.

Scans

Ultrasound

Ultrasound scans are performed either by radiographers or radiologists. The Ultrasound Department is usually next to – if not part of – X-ray, although some large obstetric departments have their own ultrasound equipment.

Nuclear medicine

Investigations using radionuclides/radioactive isotopes are performed in Nuclear Medicine, common ones being DMSA, and DTPA scans, bone scans and thyroid scans.

Some isotope tracers used in nuclear medicine

There is a strict convention for setting out isotopes. For example:

Carbon-14   or ^{14}C
Chromium-51   or ^{51}Cr

Gallium-67   or ^{67}Ga
Sellenium-75   or ^{75}Se
Technetium-99   or ^{99}Tc

The units of measurement used for radioactivity are the becquerel (Bq) which is a very small value so in practice megabecquerels (MBq) are used. The more traditional unit, the curie (Ci), is also used and values commonly seen are in MCi (millicuries) or μCi (microcuries).

The following isotopes and tracers are used in radioisotope scanning procedures of internal organs. Technetium-99 is the radionuclide most commonly used.

Radioactive isotope and symbol		Labelled substance
Carbon-14	^{14}C	lactose
		urea
Cobalt-57	^{57}Co ⎱	
Cobalt-58	^{58}Co ⎰	cyanocobalamine (DICOPAC)
Chromium-51	^{51}Cr	chromic chloride
		EDTA (ethylene diamine tetra-acetic acid)
		sodium chromate
Gallium-67	^{67}Ga	gallium citrate
Iodine-123	^{123}I	MIBG (metaiodobenzyl guanidine)
Iodine-125	^{125}I	HSA (human serum albumin)
Indium-111	^{111}In	oxine
Selenium-75	^{75}Se	SeHCAT (tauroselcholic acid)
		Scintadren
Technetium-99 m	^{99m}Tc	CERETEC (exametazime)
		DMSA (dimercapto succinate)
		DTPA (diethylene triamine pentacetic acid)
		EHIDA (etifenin)
		gluco heptonate
		HDP (oxidronate)
		hepatate II tin colloid
		hida N substituted iminodiacetic acid
		HMPAO (hexamethylipropyleneamine oxime)
		in vivo stannous chloride
		MAA (macroaggregated albumin)
		MDP (methylene diphosphonate)
		medronic acid
		MAG 3 (mercaptoacetyl-triglycine)
		pertechnetate (TcO$_4$)
		re-sulphide
Thallium-201	^{201}Tl	thallous chloride
Xenon-133	^{133}Xe	xenon gas

Computerized (axial) tomography

The CAT or CT scanner produces an image of tissue density in a complete cross-section of the body being scanned.

Magnetic resonance imaging

Magnetic resonance seans are a fairly new form of imaging that uses powerful magnets to produce detailed pictures of the body. Increasingly they are used in the investigation of the central nervous system in patients with cancer.

X-rays

X-rays form an important part of an investigation to establish a correct diagnosis. Plain X-rays of any part of the body may be taken. The following are some of the more common ones:

Type	Area of body
chest X-ray (CXR)	X-ray for chest and heart conditions but often performed as a routine procedure. It will show scarring from previous TB etc.
Mammogram	X-ray examination of breast tissue.
Pelvimetry	X-rays of the pelvis (in late pregrancy) to measure the pelvic outlet.
Orthopantomograms (OPT)	X-rays of teeth.

Some examinations require specialized techniques such as inserting 'dye' to highlight certain structures by contrast. Examples of these are:

Type	Area of body
barium swallow	detects abnormality in the oesophagus.
barium meal	examines the stomach and small intestine.
barium enema	shows up abnormalities in the colon.
intravenous pyelogram (IVP)	highlights the urinary tract.
intravenous urogram (IVU)	highlights the bladder.
micturating cystogram	a bladder examination.
cholangiogram	X-rays the gall bladder and bile duct.
cholecystogram	X-rays the gall bladder.
myelogram	spinal cord examination.
sialogram	X-ray of the salivary glands.
radiculogram	a form of spinal cord X-ray.
tomogram	X-ray of selected layers of the body.

Chapter 8
Drugs

This chapter outlines very briefly some of the different types of drugs and the conditions in which they may be used. The secretary is reminded that she should have the *British National Formulary* to hand for reference and to use this to check spelling and any other queries.

Conventions

Drugs may be called by their generic (non-proprietary) name or their proprietary (trade) name. For example, diazepam (generic name) is probably more familiar as Valium (one of its proprietary names). It is usual to write the proprietary name with an initial capital letter but not the generic name.

All drugs must be prescribed by a qualified doctor and dispensed in the presence of another person (who is not the patient).

Drugs have specific actions on various systems of the body and some can be listed under these headings (see also Chapter 5).

Organ systems and some commonly prescribed drugs

Musculoskeletal system

- **Anticholinergic drugs** are given to enhance voluntary and involuntary muscle and are commonly used to treat urinary frequency and unstable bladder.
- **Antirheumatic agents** drugs used in rheumatic diseases and gout may be anti-inflammatory analgesics such as aspirin and the salicylates; other non-steroidal anti-inflammatory drugs (often referred to as NSAIDS); corticosteroids, drugs which affect the rheumatic disease process such as penicillamine; allopurinal which may be used as a prophylactic drug in gout.

Cardiovascular system

- **Antiarrhythmic drugs** These are used in irregularities of the heart. A common one is digoxin.

- **Anticoagulant drugs** are given for the prevention or treatment of postoperative thrombosis and deep vein thrombosis (DVT). Heparin is given for immediate treatment of a thrombosis, before starting the patient on warfarin.

  Anticoagulants are also used to prevent thrombi forming on prosthetic heart valves, and the drug used is usually warfarin.
- **Beta-adrenoceptor blocking drugs** (beta-blockers) are used in the treatment of hypertension, some arrhythmias, to relieve angina, migraine and thyrotoxicosis.

  Two common examples are propranolol (Inderal), and atenolol (Tenormin).
- **Cardiac glycosides** are used in the treatment of heart failure and digoxin is the drug widely used.
- **Centrally-acting antihypertensive drugs** Aldomet is one example of the proprietary drug-containing methyldopa.
- **Diuretics** are drugs which help to eliminate excess fluids (causing tissue swelling or oedema) usually in heart conditions. They are also given in cases of hypertension.
- **Fibrinolytic drugs** e.g., streptokinase, can break up thrombi and may be used in clot in the lung (pulmonary embolism), heart attacks and any other life threatening venous thrombosis.
- **Lipid-lowering drugs** are used in some patients with high blood fats (cholesterol and triglycerides). Such patients are at risk of heart disease.
- **Vasodilators** are used in angina and heart failure. There are also peripheral and cerebral dilators of blood vessels too.

  Glyceryl trinitrate (GTN) is the drug most commonly used for quick relief in angina. Small tablets are placed under the tongue for effect. Isosorbide mononitrate is a common drug used for prevention (prophylaxis) and treatment of angina.

Respiratory system

- **Anticholinergic bronchodilators** may be used in chronic bronchitis and asthma. A common one is Slo-phyllin.
- **Antihistamines** are administered for allergic disorders such as hay fever and urticaria. A common one is Triludan.
- **Antitussives** can be cough suppressants, expectorants or compound mixtures. Linctus codeine, Benylin and Actifed are examples.
- **Bronchodilators** are given for asthma/wheezy conditions, usually as an inhalant.

  Salbutamol in the form of Ventolin is widely used, as is Bricanyl.

  Devices for inhalation are nebulizers, rotahalers and volumatics.
- **Corticosteroids** are given for the treatment of asthma orally and by inhalation. Examples of commonly used inhalants are Becotide and Pulmicort.

Central nervous system

- **Analgesics** are prescribed for pain relief and many preparations are available.

    Aspirin, paracetamol or codeine preparations are prescribed for mild to moderate pain and some compound preparations containing all three drugs are available.

    Narcotic analgesics are prescribed for moderate to severe pain; morphine and pethidine are examples.
- **Anticonvulsants** are used in epilepsy and febrile convulsions.

    Commonly used drugs are phenytoin (Epanutin), carbamazepine (Tegretol), phenobarbitone and sodium valproate.
- **Antiemetic drugs** are used in motion sickness, Menière's disease and other abnormalities of the labyrinth in the ear, postural vertigo, severe vomiting in pregnancy and vomiting caused by cytotoxic drugs or radiotherapy. There are different drugs depending on the cause of the vomiting and vertigo.
- **Antipsychotic drugs** are given in schizophrenia, some behavioural or manic disturbances and in some cases of agitation, especially in the elderly.
- **Anxiolytics** are given to relieve anxiety states. There are many different drugs in this category—including a group of drugs, known as the benzodiazepines, of which diazepam (Valium) is perhap, the best known.
- **Hypnotics** are given to induce sleep.
- **Other neurological drugs** are prescribed for, for example, parkinsonism which is a neurological disorder characterized by hypokinesia (abnormally deficient motor function), tremor and rigidity. There are also specific drugs for chorea, tics, tremor and related disorders.

Gastrointestinal system

- **Antacids** are used for indigestion (dyspepsia) caused by acidity. Some common antacids are magnesium trisilicate ('mis. mag. tri') and sodium bicarbonate.
- **Antidiarrhoeal drugs** may contain chalk, kaolin, morphine, opium or codeine phosphate.
- **Antispasmodics** are used in intestinal disorders characterized by muscle spasm such as irritable bowel syndrome. These drugs usually contain atropine sulphate or belladonna.
- **Laxatives** are prescribed for constipation, but they are 'addictive'. They are also given before some X-ray procedures such as barium enema or intravenous pyelogram.
- **Rectal-soothing agents** the drugs may be contained in the form of a suppository, commonly Anusol suppositories for haemorrhoids.
- **Ulcer-healing drugs** cimetidine (Tagamet), and ranitidine (Zantac) are two well-known ones.

Endocrine system

- **Antithyroid drugs** are used in the treatment of thyrotoxicosis, the most common one being carbimazole (Neo-mercazole).
- **Corticosteroids** are given in many different conditions such as asthma, ulcerative colitis, rheumatoid disorders, skin diseases, and some malignant tumours. Common corticosteroid drugs are betamethasone, dexamethasone and prednisolone.

  Patients on long-term steroid therapy have to carry a special card because of the dangers in stopping the drug abruptly; in cases of illness or operation the dose may have to be increased.
- **Drugs used in diabetes mellitus** are insulin preparations (human or animal) or oral hypoglycaemic drugs to lower the blood sugar, such as tolbutamide.
- **Pituitary hormone** such as clomiphene citrate (Clomid) is used in some cases of female infertility.

  A pituitary growth hormone may be used in cases of short stature in children with delayed puberty.
- **Sex hormones** male sex hormones: common drug is methyltestosterone.

  Female sex hormones: two groups are the oestrogens and progestogens.

  Anabolic steroids: their use is now banned in competitive sport but medically they may be used for a form of anaemia or debilitating disease, and in some cases of malignancy.
- **Thyroid hormones** are used in hypothyroidism (myxoedema), lymphadenoid goitre and thyroid cancer.

Infections and malignant disease

Infections

- **Antibiotics** are used to treat bacterial infections and are not effective against viruses. Some antibiotics are more effective against organisms in certain parts of the body (such as the urinary or the respiratory tract) and are therefore used more frequently for infections in those areas.

  There are many different groups of antibiotics, such as the penicillins, sulphonamides and tetracyclines.

  A few viral infections such as herpes virus may be treated with antiviral drugs (e.g. acyclovir).
- **Antifungal drugs** are used in fungal infections. A common one is caused by *candida albicans* (candidiasis, also known as monilia or thrush). Treatment in this case is often with Canesten.
- **Antihelminthics** are used for the treatment of worms.
- **Antiprotozoal drugs** are used for such infections as malaria and other mainly tropical diseases.

Malignant disease and immunosuppressants

- **Cytotoxic** drugs are used in cancer chemotherapy, and may be referred to as chemotherapy or just 'chemo'.
- **Immunosuppressant drugs** are used to prevent organ transplant rejection.

Abbreviations and terms used on prescriptions or in patients' notes

ac	before meals
bd	twice a day
mane	morning
nocte	night
od	once daily
pc	after meals
prn	when necessary
qds or qid	four times a day
R_x	let it be made or 'take thou' (R stands for recipe)
sos	if necessary
stat	at once
tds or tid	three times a day
sliding scale	dose adjusted to patient's requirements

Common methods of administering drugs and nutrients

Drugs

There are a number of different ways to administer drugs, by:

- inhalation – breathing in
- injection
  - into muscle — IM (intramuscularly)
  - into a vein — IV (intravenously)
  - under the skin — SC (subcutaneously)
- insertion into
  - the rectum — pr (per rectum) as suppositories
  - the vagina — pv (per vaginam) as pessaries
- inunction – rubbing in
- mouth — PO (per oral)
- topical application – applied locally.

Nutrients

Food may be given as:

- enteral nutrition – directly into the gastrointestinal tract via the mouth, nasogastric tube or gastrostomy.

- parenteral nutrition – any means other than through the alimentary canal, e.g. intravenous administration via a central venous catheter, directly into the bloodstream.

Units

Drugs may be prescribed in doses using the following units:

ng	nanogram	10^{-9} of a gram
mcg⎫	microgram	10^{-6} of a gram
µg ⎬		
mg	milligram	one thousandth of a gram
g	gram	
kg	kilogram	one thousand grams

Volumes
ml	millilitre	one thousandth of a litre
l	litre	one thousand millilitres

Units
U	unit
IU	International Unit

Notes
All units are 'singular' – i.e. ml not mls.
Microgram should always be spelt out in full.
Millilitres replace the now obsolete ccs.

Part III
Terminology for General Medicine and Surgery

Chapter 9
General Medical Terminology

The terminology outlined in this chapter will be found throughout all branches of medicine. It is important for all medical secretaries to be familiar with it. The chapter is set out with the typing of general medical summaries in mind.

Summaries and clinical procedure

When patients are admitted to hospital, the receiving doctor carries out a systematic enquiry and examination of the patient – and then reaches a tentative diagnosis. When summaries are dictated for typing the diagnosis usually comes first.

For the purposes of this chapter, we will look at the terminology likely to be used when the doctor is admitting a patient. The order of procedures is:

- patient's condition on arrival/admission
- organ systems enquiry with regards to symptoms
- past medical history
- physical examination
- investigations
- tentative diagnosis
- treatment
- follow-up.

Words used in general observation of patients

Some terms	Meaning
ataxic	lack of muscle co-ordination (may be cerebellar or truncal ataxia).
cachectic	thin, ill looking.
cyanosed	blue-looking through lack of oxygen.
dysphasic	impaired speech.
dyspnoeic	difficult and laboured breathing.
ecchymoses	large bruises (*adj.* ecchymotic).
facies	face, general expression.
jaundiced	yellow-coloured due to bile pigment in the skin and mucous membranes.

Some terms	*Meaning*
orthopnoeic	difficult breathing except in upright position.
petechia	red spot caused by bleeding in the skin.
plethoric	red florid complexion.
purpura	purplish or brownish discoloration caused by haemorrhage under skin.
telangiectasis	spot caused by dilated capillary (spider naevus).

Recording signs and symptoms

The patient is questioned about signs and symptoms experienced in the different systems of the body.

You will find organ system abbreviations used in the patients' notes (e.g. RS; CVS etc) but they are spelt out in full here, with some of the more unfamiliar words that may be used listed. (The order of the organ systems reflects the doctor's methodological line of enquiry.)

Central nerous system (CNS)

diplopia	double vision.
photophobia	abnormal intolerance to light.
syncope	fainting.
vertigo	giddiness, loss of balance.

Cardiovascular system (CVS)

angina pectoris	pain in the chest due to lack of blood and oxygen to the heart muscle.
claudication	pain in the legs on walking a certain distance.
paroxysmal nocturnal dyspnoea (PND)	attacks of breathlessness at night.
paroxysmal tachycardia	palpitations.
transient ischaemic attack (TIA)	transient deficiency of blood supply to the brain due to constriction of blood vessels; can affect limbs, speech or cause blackouts.

Respiratory system (RS)

epistaxis	nose bleeding.
haemoptysis	coughing up blood.
sinusitis	infection of the sinuses.
sputum or phlegm	may be purulent or mucoid.

Gastrointestinal system (GIS)

defaecation	evacuation of the bowels.
dysphagia	difficulty in swallowing.
haematemesis	vomiting up blood.
melaena	passage of dark tarry stools containing changed blood.

Some terms	*Meaning*

Urinary system (US)

dysuria	pain in passing urine.
haematuria	blood in the urine.
micturition	act of passing urine (to micturate).
nocturia	excessive passing of urine at night.

Endocrine system (ES)

hirsutism	excessive body hair.
menses	periods.
LMP	last menstrual period.
PMB or PM bleeding	postmenopausal bleeding.
polydipsia	excessive thirst.
polyuria	passing excessive amount of urine.
pruritis	itching.

Recording physical examination of patients

Words which may be used:

Eye examination

acuity	clarity of vision.
exophthalmos	forward protrusion of the eyeballs.
hemianopia	defective vision or blindness in half the field of vision.
icteric sclera	yellow discoloration of the white of the eye.
nystagmus	involuntary rapid movement of the eyeball.
optic fundi	fundi of the eye.
papilloedema	swelling of the optic papilla within the eyeball.
ptosis	drooping upper eyelid.
retinopathy	non-inflammatory disease of the retina.

Neck examination

cervical nodes	lymph glands in the neck. (Other sites of lymph glands are supra-clavicular, axillary, epitrochlear or inguinal.)
JVP	jugular venous pressure – may be raised/not raised.
lymphadenopathy	swollen lymph glands.
stiffness or rigidity	
trachea central or deviated	
thyroid nodule	goitre.

Throat

fauces	passage from mouth to pharynx, may be described as red or infected.

Some terms	Meaning

Chest

Areas
apical
costophrenic
diaphragmatic
intercostal
mediastinal
precordial
retrosternal
sternal

Findings on
auscultation (listening)
basal creps (crepitations)
bruit
crackles
rales.
rhonchi
wheezes, inspiratory or expiratory.

heart murmurs — pan systolic, flow, diastolic, soft and harsh.

pulse — sinus rhythm, sinus arrhythmia, dysrhythmia, paroxysmal atrial fibrillation, atrial or ventricular flutter, tachycardia (fast) bradycardia (slow) and irregularly/irregular

HS — heart sounds, I, II, III or IV

Abdomen

Areas
epigastric
hypogastric
hypochondrium (left and right)
iliac fossa left and right (LIF and RIF)
McBurney's point
pubic
suprapubic
umbilical.

Findings on palpation:
ascites — fluid in the abdominal cavity.
hepatomegaly — enlarged liver.
hepatosplenomegaly — liver and spleen enlarged.
inguinal nodes — glands in the groin.
rebound tenderness — signs of inflammation.
   guarding
splenomegaly — enlarged spleen.
pr (per rectum) — rectal examination.
pv (per vaginam) — vaginal examination.

Hands

clubbing — changes in the soft tissue around the ends of the fingers (terminal phalanges).

Some terms	*Meaning*
Dupuytren's contracture	shrinkage of tissues in the palm causing finger to flex.
koilonychia	mis-shapen nails.
palmar erythema	redness of palms.
tremor	trembling.

Legs

DVT	deep vein thrombosis.
oedematous	abnormally large amount of fluid in the tissues.
reflexes	Kernig's sign, Babinski's sign, plantars (up going/down going), knee jerks, ankle jerks.
thrombophlebitis	inflammation of vein with clot.
varicosities	varicose veins.

Blood pressure

systolic and diastolic – e.g. 140/90 mm of mercury (Hg) (mmHg).
(140 systolic over 90 mmHg diastolic)

hypertension	high blood pressure.
hypotension	low blood pressure.
normotensive	normal blood pressure.

Peripheral pulses

carotid
dorsalis pedis
femoral
popliteal
posterior tibial
brachial
radial.

Possible conditions and their meanings featuring in the diagnosis

The following list is intended to convey only the most usual diagnoses of patients in the general medical wards. Many neurological and endocrine diseases, as well as rarer illnesses and syndromes, have not been included. Some diseases caused by microorganisms are listed in Chapter 16.

Some terms	*Meaning*

Blood conditions

anaemia	can be aplastic, autoimmune, β-thalassaemia, erythroblastic, haemolytic, hypochromic, hypoplastic, icterohaemolytic, macrocytic, megaloblastic, pernicious, sickle cell, sideroblastic, and spherocytic.

Some terms	Meaning
leukaemia	may be myeloid, lymphoid, myeloblastic, monocytic, lymphocytic, lymphatic. Myeloproliferative disorder/syndrome may refer to a form of leukaemia or other serious blood disease.
lymphoma	any neoplastic disorder of the lymphoid tissue. May be Hodgkin's disease or non-Hodgkin's lymphomas. The latter include Burkitt's lymphoma.
myeloma	tumour formed of cells found in the bone marrow. May be known as a plasmacytoma, or multiple myeloma.
polycythaemia rubra vera (PRV)	an abnormal increase in the number of red blood cells.
thrombocytopenic purpura	a bleeding disorder – causing extensive bruising – due to seriously reduced numbers of platelets in the blood.

Central nervous system

CVA	cerebrovascular accident (a stroke).
epilepsy	characterized by (seizures) fits which may be *grand mal* (major fit) or *petit mal* (momentary loss of consciousness).
Berry aneurysm	leaking aneurysm in the brain. Aneurysm is a sac formed by dilation of artery or vein.
multiple sclerosis (MS)	progressive degenerative disease of the myelin sheath of nervous system and spine causing paralysis.
Parkinson's disease	Progressive, degenerative disease characterized by fine resting tremor.
subarachnoid haemorrhage	bleeding into subarachnoid space (see Ch. 5) of brain.

Cardiovascular system

artrial fibrillation (AF)	cardiac arrhythmia.
atrial flutter	form of cardiac arrhythmia.
bacterial endocarditis (SBE)	subacute bacterial endocardition, a serious infection of the endocardium.
congestive cardiac failure (CCF)	abnormal circulatory congestion caused by blockage of the heart's ventricles and sodium and water retention by the kidneys.
cor pulmonale	serious condition with right ventricular heart failure.

Some terms	*Meaning*
extra systoles	ectopics, ectopic (extra) beats.
heart block	partial or complete: 1st, 2nd or 3rd degree.
ischaemic heart disease	deficiency of blood to the heart.
mitral stenosis	narrowing of the left atrioventricular orifice (mitral orifice).
mitral incompetence	defective mitral valve causing blood to flow from left ventricle back into left atrium.
myocardial infarction (MI)	coronary thrombosis: heart attack.
pericarditis	inflammation of the pericardium.
ventricular ectopics (VEs)	an extra heart beat, normal in healthy children and young adults but indicative of disease in an older person.

Respiratory system

alveolitis	inflammation of the alveoli of the lung.
asthma	disorder characterized by recurrent episodes of wheezing and severe breathlessness.
aspergillosis	disease caused by the organism Aspergillus (a type of fungus).
atelectasis	collapsed or airless state of the lung.
bronchiectasis	chronic dilation of the bronchi and bronchioles with secondary infection.
bronchitis	acute or chronic (usually) inflammation of the tissue of the bronchi.
carcinoma of the lung	lung cancer.
COAD	chronic obstructive airways disease.
emphysema	loss of elasticity in the lung tissues. due to the terminal bronchioles becoming plugged with mucus.
empyema	purulent (infected) exudate in the pleural cavity.
interstitial pulmonary fibrosis	fibrous tissue in the interspaces of the lung.
pleural effusion	accumulation of fluid in the pleural space.
pneumonia	acute inflammation of the lungs.
pneumothorax	air in the pleural cavity.
pulmonary embolism (PE)	obstruction of the pulmonary artery or one of its branches by an embolus (clot or other plug).
pulmonary tuberculosis (TB)	tuberculosis of the lung, chronic disease caused by an acid-fast bacillus. *Mycobacterium tuberculosis*.

Some terms	*Meaning*

Gastroenterological conditions

achalasia	failure of oesophagus to relax when swallowing.
carcinoma of the stomach	stomach cancer.
coeliac disease (pronounced 'seeliac')	a malabsorption syndrome due to allergy to gluten in foodstuffs.
Crohn's disease	an inflammatory disease of the alimentary tract.
diverticulitis	inflammation of the small blind pouches that form in the lining and wall of the colon (diverticula).
hiatus hernia	hernia through the oesophageal hiatus of the diaphragm.
ileitis	inflammation of the ileum (distal portion of the small intestine).
irritable bowel syndrome	a psycho–gastroenterological disorder where previous or on-going emotional stress causes abdominal pain, distention and diarrohea or constipation, or both.
oesophagitis	inflammation of the lining of the oesophagus.
oesophageal reflux	'water brash'; reflux of stomach contents.
oesophageal varices	varicose veins of the lower oesophagus; may cause sudden haemorrhage.
proctitis	inflammation of the rectum.
ulcerative colitis	inflammatory disease of the colon.
ulcers duodenal, gastric, peptic	erosion of mucosal lining exposing raw areas.

Liver conditions

cirrhosis	chronic, degenerative disease of lobes of liver.
hepatitis	inflammatory condition of liver may be mild or severe and life-threatening. Many causes.
hepatitis A	a form of infectious viral hepatitis. Common in young adults who make complete recovery. Virus spread directly or by contaminated water or faeces. Also called infective hepatitis.
hepatitis B	a form of viral hepatitis transmitted by contaminated blood serum or needles. Can cause prolonged illness and death. Also called serum hepatitis.
hepatoma	tumour of the liver.

Kidney conditions

nephritis	inflammation of the kidney.

Some terms	*Meaning*
nephrotic syndrome	kidney disease especially marked by degenerative lesions of the renal tubules.
pyelitis	inflammation of the renal pelvis.
renal calculi	stones causing severe pain and shock. (renal colic)
renal failure	failure of the kidney to function – through disease or trauma. Causing toxic state and uraemia.
uraemia	high levels of urea and other waste products in the blood.

Gall bladder conditions

cholelithiasis	stones in the gall bladder which can cause severe pain (biliary colic).
cholecystitis	acute or chronic inflammation of the gall bladder.

Pancreas

diabetes mellitus	complex disorder of protein, fat and carbohydrate metabolism that is largely the result of lack (absolute or relative) of the hormone insulin.
pancreatitis	inflammatory condition of the pancreas.

Thyroid gland

hyperthyroidism	excessive activity of the gland. Also known as thyrotoxicosis or Graves' disease.
hypothyroidism	deficiency of thyroid gland activity, also known as myxoedema.

Some abbreviations and their meaning

The following are often to be found in patients' notes:

AF	atrial fibrillation.
AK	above knee.
APH	antepartum haemorrhage.
BCC	basal cell carcinoma (form of skin cancer).
BK	below knee.
BO	bowels open.
BP	blood pressure.
CBD	common bile duct.
CCF	congestive cardiac failure.
CIN	cervical intraepithelial neoplasm (refers to abnormal cervical smears), may be classed as I, II or III.
CMC	carpometocarpal (joint).

CVP	central venous pressure.
DIC	diffuse intravascular coagulation.
DIP	distal interphalangeal (joint).
DOB	date of birth.
D&V	diarrhoea and vomiting.
DU	duodenal ulcer.
ECT	electroconvulsive therapy.
ERCP	endoscopic retrograde cholangiopancreatogram.
ERPC	evacuation of retained products of conception.
EUM	external urinary meatus.
FB	foreign body.
FH	family history – or in obstetrics, fetal heart (heard).
FTA	failed to attend (DNA – did not attend used in some hospitals).
GA	general anaesthetic.
GU	gastric ulcer.
LA	local anaesthetic.
LSCS	lower segment Caesarean section.
MCP	metacarpophalangeal (joint).
MI	myocardial infarction (also mitral incompetence).
MS	multiple sclerosis (also mitral stenosis).
MTP	metatarsophalangeal (joint).
MUA	manipulation under anaesthetic.
MVD	mitral valve disease.
NAD	no appreciable disease/no abnormality detected (often written nad).
NBI	no bony injury.
NFA	no fixed abode.
NFR	not for resuscitation.
NG	new growth – tumour.
OA	osteoarthritis.
O/E	on examination.
OPD	outpatient department.
PH	past history.
PID	pelvic inflammatory disease or prolapsed intervertebral disc.
PIP	proximal interphalangeal (joint).
PMH	past medical history.
POC	products of conception.
PPH	post-partum haemorrhage.
PUO	pyrexia of unknown origin.
RA/RhA	rheumatoid arthritis.
RTA	road traffic accident.
SB	stillbirth/stillborn.
SCC	squamous cell carcinoma.
SE	systems enquiry.
SH	social history.
SI	sacroiliac (joint); also sexual intercourse.
SLE	systemic lupus erythematosis.

SOB	short of breath.
TAH	total abdominal hysterectomy.
TCC	transitional cell carcinoma (bladder).
TCI	to come in – i.e. to be admitted.
THR	total hip replacement.
TKR	total knee replacement.
TMJ	temporomandibular joint.
TPR	temperature, pulse and respiration.
TTO	to take out – usually refers to medication on discharge.
TURP	transurethral resection of prostate.
UDT	undescended testis.
URTI	upper respiratory tract infection.
UTI	urinary tract infection.
UVL	ultraviolet light.
VF	ventricular fibrillation.
VSD	ventricular septal defect.
VV	varicose veins.
XROA	X-ray on arrival (at outpatient clinic).

Some symbols, and their meaning

The following symbols, may be found in patients' notes.

△	diagnosis
#	fracture
♂	male
♀	female
−ve	negative
+ve	positive
°jaundice
°oedema	no jaundice, oedema etc.
†	dead

Chapter 10
Medical Summaries and Reports

This chapter contains sample reports on patients in general medicine, neurology, endocrinology and haematology. Some terminology used in ECGs is included, as well as examples of X-ray reports.

Meanings of medical words not previously mentioned are explained but it should be emphasized that familiarity with the general usage and spelling of many terms is of as much value as total understanding of them medically.

All drug names, should be checked for spelling in the *British National Formulary*.

Examples of medical summaries with explanations of terms used

Example 10.1   Medical summary

Diagnosis

   (1) **Ischaemic heart disease**
   (2) Slow **atrial fibrillation**
   (3) **Intermittent claudication**

History

Aged 83. Past history of exertional chest pain relieved by **GTN**. On the day of admission he had two episodes lasting an hour which were not responsive to GTN. Slightly short of breath but no sweating or nausea.

Past medical history: He has suffered from angina for two years and had a stroke affecting his right visual field a year ago. Medication on admission, nifedipine 20 mg bd, slow-release GTN, fibre gel and lactulose.

Examination

He was comfortable and not in pain. Pulse 96 irregular, BP 170/110. Apex was displaced laterally. There were no peripheral pulses palpable in his right foot; pulses were present in his left foot. He had a few basal crepitations. Abdominal examination was normal. Neurological examination revealed a right **homonymous hemianopia** only.

$\rightarrow$

> ### Investigations
>
> ECG showed left axis deviation, atrial fibrillation and left **ventricular hypertrophy** with S–T segment depression in leads V_4–V_6.
>
> *Other investigations:* Hb 16, WBC 10.3, urea 4.63, creatinine 86. Liver function tests normal and cardiac enzymes were not raised.
>
> A 24-hour tape was performed because he was noticed to have several pauses on his ECGs and this showed atrial fibrillation with numerous pauses, the longest at 2.8 seconds. He had occasional **ventricular ectopics** from one run of **trigeminy**.
>
> He has been referred to the cardiologists to see whether he needs a prophylactic pacemaker. At present he has not experienced any blackouts or dizzy spells.
>
> ### Medication on discharge
>
> > nifedipine 20 mg bd
> > isosorbide mononitrate 20 mg tds
> > aspirin 150 mg mane
> > GTN prn.
>
> ### Follow up
>
> Clinic in one month's time.

Explanation of terms used in Example 10.1

atrial fibrillation   irregular heart beats caused by rapid contractions of the atrial myocardium (muscle of the heart).

claudication   weakness of legs with cramp-like pain.

GTN   Glyceryl trinitrate (see Chapter 8 on drugs).

homonymous hemianopia   defective vision or blindness in half the visual fields of the right or left halves of both eyes.

ischaemic heart disease   deficiency of blood supply to the heart muscle due to obstruction or constriction of the coronary arteries.

trigeminy   occurrence of three pulse beats in rapid succession (ECG term).

ventricular ectopics   misplaced heart beats (ECG term).

ventricular hypertrophy   enlargement of the muscle of the ventricle.

Electrocardiogram terms

As will be seen from Example 10.1, ECG terms are frequently used in reports about patients with heart problems. An ECG will include information derived from the following leads and electrodes placed on the patient's chest:

$$I, II, III, aVR, aVL, aVF, V_1-V_6$$

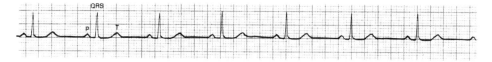

Fig. 10.1 The normal electrocardiogram: it is composed of a P wave, a QRS complex, and a T wave. (*Source* Leatham, Bull and Braimbridge 1991.)

A normal electrocardiogram is composed of a P wave, a QRS complex, and a T wave (see Fig. 10.1).

Some ECG terms commonly used might include:

artefact episodes
asystole (pause)
bigeminy/trigeminy
normal P axis
P–R interval
PSVT (paroxysmal supraventricular tachycardia)
sinus rhythm
S–T depression/episode/levels
SVE (supraventricular ectopics)
T wave inversion or flattening
VE (ventricular ectopics)

In some cases of heart irregularities, a shock may be administered to the heart to regulate the beat. This is called defibrillation.

Example 10.2   Medical summary

> ### Diagnosis
>
> Cardiac failure
>
> ### History
>
> This 73-year-old man was admitted from the clinic having become increasingly short of breath over the past 10 weeks. His ankle oedema had worsened and he complained of feeling very tired.
>
> *Past medical history*: **rheumatic fever** aged 19, **aortic regurgitation** noted. **Subacute bacterial endocarditis** aged 50, affecting the aortic valve. Complete heart block, pacemaker fitted ten years previously and reviewed eight years ago. He also suffers from **rheumatoid arthritis, gout and psoriasis.**
> $\rightarrow$

Examination

On examination he was plethoric with a slightly mooned face and bull neck. He was mildy cyanosed and had joint changes, particularly in his hands, representative of rheumatoid arthritis. His pulse was 75 regular, BP 140/90, JVP was raised 8 cm and there was a soft **diastolic murmur** representative of aortic regurgitation. Marked bilateral basal crepitations both lung bases, pitting oedema to his knees.

Progress

He was admitted so that his cardiac failure could be controlled better and any possible cause for it in terms of deteriorating heart function or valvular abnormality further investigated. An **echocardiogram** was performed but was unhelpful as the aortic valve was not identified. The mitral valve was normal and the left ventricle was dilated. Subacute endocarditis was excluded as he did not have a temperature during his admission and his blood cultures were negative.

His heart failure slowly improved throughout his admission and he was treated with **diuretics** and captopril.

On discharge an appointment was made for him to be seen for a repeat **cardiac catheterization**.

Investigations

Hb 12.6, WBC 7.1, MCV 102, B_{12} and folate normal.
ESR 40, U & Es and LFTs nad, urea 9.8 on discharge.
GGT slightly raised 80 iu/l, urate 0.68; thyroxine nad.
On his CXR, cardiac pacing wires and pacemaker noted, also the heart was markedly enlarged, especially when compared with previous films.

A pericardial effusion should be considered. Appearances in the lung fields are suggestive of congestive cardiac failure. There was some widening and blurring of the superior mediastinum possibly due to vena cava obstruction, but compatible with congestive heart failure.
His ECG showed an artificial pacemaker rhythm rate 72 with underlying **atrial flutter**. There were no acute changes.

Medication on discharge

> sulphasalazine e/c 1 g tds
> piroxicam 20 mg nocte
> frusemide 80 mg mane, 40 mg lunchtime
> captopril 25 mg tds
> prednisolone 5 mg mane
> allopurinol 100 mg od
> isosorbide mononitrate 10 mg bd

Follow-up

He will be seen again in OPD in six weeks after his cardiac catheterization.

Explanation of terms used in Example 10.2

aortic regurgitation   defect in the aortic valve allowing regurgitation of blood.

atrial flutter   a type of irregularity of the heart beat.

cardiac catheterization   heart investigation necessitating the passage of a fine tube (catheter) into the arteries to the heart.

diastolic murmur   a heart murmur heard in the diastolic phase of the cardiac cycle.

diuretics   drugs given to increase urine output and so reduce tissue swelling (oedema).

echocardiogram   a heart investigation using echoes of ultrasonic beams.

gout   a form of arthritis caused by excess uric acid in the blood.

pericardial effusion   presence of liquid in the outer covering of the heart (pericardium).

psoriasis   a skin condition.

rheumatic fever   an acute form of rheumatism which can affect the heart valves.

rheumatoid arthritis   condition affecting many different joints causing inflammation, serious deformity and disability.

subacute bacterial endocarditis   a serious condition caused by bacterial infection of the lining of the heart (endocardium).

Example 10.3   PA (posterior–anterior) erect chest radiograph summary

The **cardiac shadow is** enlarged.

A prominent **pleural effusion** is present on the left and a minimal lamella effusion on the right side.

Basal septal lines are noted particularly in the right lower zone.

Some upper lobe blood diversion is noted reflecting **raised pulmonary venous pressure**.

Calcification is seen projected over the cardiac shadow, this is probably in costal cartilage.

Impression: Appearances are those of mild **congestive cardiac failure** with **interstitial pulmonary oedema** and prominent left sided pleural effusion.

Example 10.4   Portable antero–posterior (AP) supine chest radiograph summary
Patient on ventilator in Intensive Care (intensive therapy unit or ITU)

It is not possible to assess the size of the cardiac shadow accurately on this radiograph. An endotracheal tube is noted *in situ*, the tip is approximately →

2 cm from the carina (projection of lowest tracheal cartilage) and needs to be pulled back another cm. A **venous line** is noted on the right, its tip is in the right ventricle and should be replaced in the right atrium or superior vena cava. No evidence of pleural effusions or **pneumothorax** seen. The lung fields are clear.

Explanation of terms used in Examples 10.3 and 10.4 and other chest X-rays

basal septal lines   outline of the bottom 'inner' margins of the lungs.

calcification   deposits of calcium showing up on an X-ray as opacities.

cardiac shadow   outline of the heart.

congestive cardiac failure   congestion of the circulatory system caused by heart disease.

consolidation   becoming solid, i.e. areas of lung which have become firm and inelastic.

interstitial pulmonary oedema   accumulation of fluid in the interstitial spaces of the lungs.

pleural effusion   abnormal accumulation of fluid in the interstitial and air spaces of the lungs.

pulmonary venous pressure   the pressure exerted against the walls of the pulmonary vein by the passage of blood.

Example 10.5   Neurology summary

Diagnosis

Investigation of fits.

History

This 28-year-old woman was admitted after an episode of loss of consciousness – she had awoken to find herself lying on the floor, having been incontinent of urine. A couple of weeks earlier she had been admitted to hospital after what sounds like a fit with **Todd's paralysis**. A CT brain **scan** and **lumbar puncture** at the time were reported as being normal. She has no previous history of epilepsy, head injury or migraine.

Past medical history: Nil of note. She is not on any medication, is a non-smoker and does not drink alcohol. This is her first pregnancy.

Examination

Temperature 37.3; pulse 86 and regular; BP 110/80; HS – normal with no added murmurs. Chest – clear. Abdominal palpation normal. CNS – she was fully conscious, orientated. No neck stiffness. **Pupils equally responsive to light and** examination of the fundi were normal. In the limbs there was   →

minimal weakness of the left arm and left leg. **Plantar responses were bilaterally flexor**.

Investigations

Hb. 11.7, WBC 8, platelets 181. Glucose 4.5, urea, electrolytes and calcium normal. EEG – normal.

Treatment and progress

Whilst on the ward, she was witnessed by the nursing staff to have further **grand mal** fits, usually lasting 1–2 minutes. During these episodes all her limbs were shaking and she was confused **post-ictally**. Blood glucose was estimated after some of these episodes and found to be normal. The patient was reluctant to take **anticonvulsant medication** and it was explained that the risk of further fits would be more harmful to the fetus than the drugs.

Later underlying psychological problems were discovered, including a tendency to **anorexia nervosa**.

Explanation of terms used in Example 10.5

anorexia nervosa   a serious condition in which the patient refuses to eat and becomes emaciated and physically ill. Associated with underlying psychological problems.

anticonvulsant medication   drugs given to prevent fits.

CT scan   computerized tomographic picture highlighting different densities of cross-sectioned parts of the body.

epilepsy   a group of neurological disorders characterized by seizures. Most cases of no known cause.

grand mal   major epileptic fit.

ictal   pertaining to epileptic seizure (or a stroke).

lumbar puncture   tapping the subarachnoid space in the lumbar vertebrae of spine to obtain cerebrospinal fluid (csf) for analysis.

plantar response   reflex flexing of toe, when outer surface of sole of foot stroked firmly.

pupil equally responsive to light   neurological observation test carried out by nursing and medical staff at specific intervals. Light shone into patient's eyes and reaction of pupil noted. Gives indication of neurological state.

Example 10.6   Neurology summary – letter form

Thank you for referring this gentleman who has had longstanding neurological problems since a child. This has throughout involved difficulty in walking and it is this same problem which has become worse of late. Over the last few years he has had increasing problems with balance, with

→

anxiety and with a desire to rush at everything. Since a course of physiotherapy he has shown some marked improvement.

On examination he has a **horizontal nystagmus** to both left and right, greater to the left. He has an **intention tremor,** fully co-ordinated **heel/shin,** positive **Romberg's** and a broad-based gait. Reflexes are normal and equal. **Plantars down-going** and tone is normal. **Fundi** are normal.

It seems likely that this is some form of **congenital cerebellar dysfunction,** but I have also ordered various blood tests and a CT scan today, to exclude other possible causes for his deterioration. I will see him again in two months.

Explanation of terms used in Example 10.6

congenital cerebellar dysfunction   an abnormality from birth of the part of the brain (cerebellum) concerned with both coarse and fine movement, and balance.

fundi   the back of the eye – visualized with an ophthalmoscope. Indicates neurological state.

heel/shin   a test of the co-ordination where the patient runs the heel down the opposite shin.

intention tremor   tremor on specific movement, such as picking up a glass.

nystagmus   involuntary rhythmical movements of the eye(s). Indicative of various neurological disorders.

plantar reflex   a response in the big toe obtained by stroking the sole of the foot. Normal is for the toe to flex down (withdraw). It is abnormal if the big toe points up (extends).

Romberg's sign   swaying of the body or falling when standing with the feet close together and the eyes closed.

Example 10.7   Endocrinology summary

Diagnosis

Diabetic **ketoacidosis**

History

This 76-year-old man who is a known **insulin-dependent diabetic** was admitted with **polyuria, polydipsia** and drowsiness.

He had only recently been discharged from the ward, and on the day of admission felt too ill to inject his own insulin.

Therapy: He is normally on Mixtard 16 units in the morning and 20 units in the evening.

$\rightarrow$

Examination

Temperature 36.5. He appeared very dehydrated, pulse rate 110, blood pressure 110/60. There was a soft systolic murmur on **auscultation** and the chest appeared clear. The abdomen was soft and non-tender. On neurological examination he was very drowsy but there was no evidence of **focal neuropathy**.

Investigations

BM Stix showed a level of 44 mmol/l, urinalysis showed glucose + + + + and a large amount of **ketonuria**. This was confirmed by the laboratory sugar of 55, sodium 129, potassium 6.8, bicarbonate 3, urea 17.8. MSU – nad.

Progress

He was treated with potassium, fluids and insulin replacement. It was noted that his insulin injection technique was not perfect but improved on re-education.

Medication on discharge

He was discharged on Mixtard 20 units bd and ranitidine 150 mg nocte.

Follow-up

He will be reviewed in the diabetic clinic.

Explanation of terms used in Example 10.7

auscultation   art of listening to sounds within the body – usually with a stethoscope.

BM stix   Proprietary means of monitoring sugar content in the blood obtained from a pinprick and applied to an impregnated stick. Result then read off.

focal neuropathy   focus of functional disturbance or pathological change in the peripheral nervous system.

insulin-dependent diabetic   patient with diabetes mellitus demanding stabilization with injections of insulin.

ketoacidosis   abnormal increase in hydrogen ions and ketones in the body's tissue.

ketonuria   excessive ketones in the urine. Ketones become present when carbohydrate metabolism is faulty. It is a feature of uncontrolled diabetes: the patient is in diabetic coma or in danger of it.

polydipsia   excessive thirst.

polyuria   passing excessive quantities of urine.

Example 10.8   Endocrinology summary – letter form

I reviewed this lady with **hyperthyroid disease** in the clinic today. She is much improved since her first presentation although she is still quite anxious. Her most recent T_4 level was 124 which is within the normal range and I think some of her anxiety is due to stress at home.

She was clinically **euthyroid** with a pulse of 84, although she has been on **beta-blockers**. There was no appreciable tremor.

I reduced her carbimazole to 10 mg bd and have also suggested she should reduce her propranolol to 40 mg bd. We will review her in four weeks' time with a repeat of her thyroid tests.

Explanation of terms used in Example 10.8

T_4 thyroxine level in the blood.

beta-blockers   drugs used in the treatment of hypertension, thyrotoxicosis and heart arrhythmias (see Chapter 8).

euthyroid   normal thyroid balance.

hyperthyroid disease   excessive activity of the thyroid (also known as thyrotoxicosis or Graves' disease).

Example 10.9   Thyroid scan report (nuclear medicine department)

The examination was performed with 87 MBq of technetium-99^m-labelled pertechnetate. The relevant uptake and trapping of pertechnetate is 5.3% of injected dose at 20 minutes (normal range 0.5–3%)

There is homogeneous uptake throughout both lobes of the thyroid with uptake in the pyramidal lobes.

The appearances are consistent with Graves' disease.

A list of these radionucleotides and isotope tracers and abbreviations is included in Chapter 7.

Example 10.10   Haematology summary

Diagnosis

Multiple myeloma

History

This lady with multiple myeloma was admitted because of pain around her chest and loss of power. $\rightarrow$

As you know, her myeloma became resistant to **melphalan**. Her **paraprotein** level was increasing and she became **hypercalcaemic** and anaemic. her ESR was increasing and also her β_2 – microglobulin.

Investigations

On admission her haemoglobin was 12.6, white cells 9.4, platelets 119, and the **ESR** was 102. The blood urea was 9.7, creatinine 132, and calcium level 3.39.

Treatment and progress

The hypercalcaemia was treated by intravenous fluids, **diuretics** and high doses of **prednisolone**. As the myeloma had become resistant to melphalan she was given a combination of **chemotherapy** which consisted of melphalan 10 mg daily for five days, cyclophosphamide 500 mg iv stat, BiCNU (Carmustine) 40 mg iv stat and vincristine 1.5 mg iv stat. These were given with **allopurinol**.

During her stay in hospital she gradually improved, the pain lessened and the calcium level returned to normal. As a result of the chemotherapy she became **thrombocytopenic**. The platelet count went down to 26 but there were no bleeding problems.

She was discharged twelve days after admission when her appetite was improving and her blood count acceptable.

Follow-up

The course of the chemotherapy is usually for two weeks and we plan to repeat it within five weeks. She will be reviewed next week in Outpatients.

Explanation of terms used in Example 10.10

allopurinol drugs commonly given for gout but also used with cytotoxic drugs.

chemotherapy normally used to denote cancer chemotherapy but sometimes used to refer to antibiotic treatment.

diuretics drugs given to increase the urine output to reduce fliud accumulated in tissues.

ESR erythrocyte sedimentation rate: the rate at which red blood cells, will separate out from blood plasma when left to stand. Indicative of many things, including active disease process.

hypercalcaemic high calcium level in the blood.

melphalan a cytotoxic drug used in cancer treatment.

multiple myeloma malignant neoplasm of the plasma cells arising in the bone marrow and characterized by bone pain and skeletal destruction.

paraprotein immunoglobulin produced by tumour plasma cells in diseases such as myeloma.

prednisolone a corticosteroid drug.
thrombocytopenic decrease in the number of clotting blood cells (platelets).
IV intravenous

Example 10.11   Haematology summary

Diagnosis

> **Thrombocythaemia**

History

This lady with previous **thrombocythaemia** was admitted for blood transfusion because she developed **pancytopenia**

Investigations

Her haemoglobin was 4.7, white cells 2.8, and platelets 35

Treatment and progress

A bone marrow aspiration was performed which showed **aplastic** marrow secondary to previous **bulsulphan** therapy.

She was given six units of packed cells which was uneventful and she was then discharged. She is on no medication and we will review her again in the Haematology Clinic.

Explanation of terms used in Example 10.11

aplastic a failure of development of normal cells, tissues, etc., suffering from aplasia.
busulphan cytotoxic drug used in cancer chemotherapy.
pancytopenia deficiency of all cell elements in blood.
thrombocythaemia abnormal increase in the number of circulating blood platelets.

Chapter 11
Surgical Terminology and Reports

This chapter contains samples of surgical summaries, abdominal X-ray reports, femoral arteriograms and examples of general surgical operations. It is particularly valuable, therefore, to the general surgery secretary and to the secretary working in X-ray.

Tumours

As quite a large number of surgical procedures involve the resection of tumours, some knowledge of terminology used regarding them is useful. Tumours may be benign (innocent) or malignant (likely to spread near (locally) or far (distally)). As shown in Chapter 6 the suffix '-oma' means tumour. There are many different forms such as adenoma, chondroma, epithelioma, granuloma, haemangioma, lipoma, melanoma, neuroma, osteoma and papilloma. The prefix indicates the type of tumour – e.g. haem- to do with blood; lip- to do with fat.

Carcinomas and sarcomas

These are malignant tumours which may spread locally or by secondary deposits called metastases (or 'secondaries'). When a patient has secondaries he or she may be said to be suffering from metastatic disease and when tumours are multiple and widespread the term 'carcinomatosis' is sometimes used. When examined histologically malignant tumours may be described as being well differentiated, poorly differentiated, invasive or infiltrating. Tumours which are described as '*in situ*' have not spread. Dysplasia and dyskaryosis are abnormalities of cells which can be precancerous.

As well as the tumours already mentioned there are cysts of all types, a common one being a sebaceous or epidermal cyst. Other examples of growths are warts, which can be of viral origin, naevi (single naevus) keratosis (a horny growth) – commonly seborrhoeic keratosis – and polyps which in general surgery are frequently found in the colon and rectum.

Some abbreviations regarding tumours are found in the list at the end of Chapter 9.

Examples of surgical summaries with explanations of terms used

Example 11.1   Surgical summary

Diagnosis

    (1) Left **inguinal hernia**
    (2) Acute **urinary retention**
    (3) **Haematemesis**

Operation

    Left inguinal herniorrhaphy
    Upper GI endoscopy
    TURP

Routine admission for left inguinal hernia repair. The patient is a known diabetic on gliclazide. On clinical examination he was found to have a very large prostate gland and was therefore **catheterized** preoperatively and the catheter left *in situ*.

Procedure

Left inguinal herniorrhaphy. Surgeon Mr Brown Anaesthetist Dr Smith.

Postoperatively, the patient progressed well and the catheter was removed on the second day. As he appeared to be passing urine satisfactorily he was discharged home.

Progress

However he was re-admitted in acute urinary retention two days later and catheterization revealed a residual urinary volume of 1200 ml. He also admitted to having **coffee-ground vomit** although at the time his haemoglobin was 13.4. In view of the possible history of haematemesis he was referred for endoscopy which showed a grade 2 **oesophagitis** with normal stomach and mild **duodenitis**. He was commenced on antireflux therapy. A trial without **catheter** failed to relieve his urinary retention and he therefore underwent a TURP.

He made an uneventful postoperative recovery following this and was discharged home.

Follow-up

To be reviewed in Outpatients.

Drugs on discharge

    atenolol 100 mg daily
    gliclazide 160 mg mane and 8 mg nocte
    Gastrocote 10 ml qds
    ranitidine 300 mg nocte.

Explanation of terms used in Example 11.1

catheter   tube for withdrawing fluids. Common urinary catheters are Foley and Malecot.

catheterized   having a tube in the bladder in order to empty it.

coffee-ground vomit   description of vomit containing dark blood mixed with the stomach contents.

duodenitis   inflammation of the duodenum.

haematemesis   vomiting blood.

herniorrhaphy   repair of a hernia.

inguinal hernia   hernia in the region of the groin. Other common hernias are femoral, umbilical, paraumbilical, ventral and incisional (at the site of an operation scar). Hernias may be described as being reducible or irreducible. Irreducible hernias may strangulate causing intestinal obstruction when a loop of bowel becomes trapped. If this bowel is not released quickly it may become gangrenous and have to be resected and the remaining bowel anastomosed (joining one tube or vessel to another).

oesophagitis   inflammation of the oesophagus often caused when the gastric contents reflux back into the oesophagus.

upper GI endoscopy   examining the upper gastrointestinal tract with the aid of an endoscope.

urinary retention   inability to pass urine.

TURP   Transurethral resection of the prostate grand. Operation done via a cystoscope to resect the prostate gland. No abdominal incision is therefore necessary and the patient does not have to stay long in hospital.

Example 11.2   Surgical summary

Diagnosis

Adenocarcinoma of the colon
Ovarian cyst.

Operation

Anterior resection of rectum and right **oophorectomy**.

History

This lady was admitted with a history of change of bowel habit, weight loss and passage of blood and mucus per rectum. She had no previous medical history of note.

$\rightarrow$

Examination and investigations

On examination, she was felt to have a mass in her left iliac fossa and **sigmoidoscopy** showed an obstructing **lesion** at 14 cm. Her blood picture, liver function tests and chest X-ray were all normal.

Procedure

She underwent an anterior resection and was found to have a bulky tumour of the sigmoid colon adherent to the pelvis on the left side and a right ovary which was cystic.

Histology of the bowel tumour showed it to be a Dukes' B adenocarcinoma with adequate excision. The ovarian cyst was a benign **serous** cystadenoma.

Progress

She made an uneventful postoperative recovery apart from slight frequency and **dysuria** when her catheter was removed. She was given a course of antibiotics and discharged home.

Follow-up

She will be reviewed in Outpatient's in six weeks' time.

Explanation of terms used in Example 11.2

adenocarcinoma   malignant tumour of the colon.

dysuria   pain on passing urine.

lesion   any pathological disturbance. Often used to refer to a tumour.

oophorectomy   removal of an ovary.

serous   pertaining to or resembling serum – i.e. clear fluid normally from blood.

sigmoidoscopy   examination of the bowel with a sigmoidoscope, often performed in the outpatient clinic.

Example 11.3   Surgical summary

Diagnosis

   Abdominal aortic aneurysm

Operation

   Abdominal aortic Dacron straight graft.

History

This 75-year-old patient presented with a history of left calf **claudication** but this did not limit him to any severe extent. He had no history of rest pain or any **paraesthesia** in his legs. The patient had a previous history of chest pain but had no true history of angina but there was a probable history of **amaurosis fugax** in the past.

Examination and investigations

On examination he was found to have an abdominal aortic aneurysm which clinically measured about 5 cm. He had no pulses below his left **femoral**. His posterior **tibial Doppler pressure** was 90 on the left compared to 135 on the right with brachial pressure of 140 mmHg. A right perfemoral arteriogram was attempted; however, there was considerable difficulty in catheterizing the right femoral artery and therefore a left perfemoral arteriogram was performed which showed a long superficial femoral artery block with refilling of the **popliteal** via **collaterals** and there was a good distal run off in the left leg. His left profunda was patent. Ultrasound of the abdominal aorta confirmed a maximum diameter of 5.9 cm. As this patient was able to walk for an indefinite distance without actually stopping, his claudication certainly was not a major problem and it was decided his abdominal aortic aneurysm should be dealt with first.

Progress

The patient made an excellent recovery and was discharged home on low-dose aspirin to be reviewed in the surgical Outpatients.

Follow-up

On review at the clinic his abdominal wound was well healed with no evidence of sepsis, herniation or **haematoma**. Both his feet were warm and pink and there was no evidence of acute **ischaemic** changes. His left foot was well **perfused**. His graft is working well. I have requested full blood count, urine electrolytes and have advised him to continue with the low dose aspirin.

We will see him again in six weeks' time.

Explanation of terms used in Example 11.3

amaurosis fugax sudden transitory partial blindness without apparent lesion of the eye.

aneurysm sac formed by dilation of a blood vessel. The aorta is the largest artery in the body so an aneurysm in this site is particularly serious – a ruptured abdominal aortic aneurysm is often fatal. Great advances have been made in arterial surgery. Nowadays synthetic grafts can be inserted so that the abnormal lower aorta can be replaced.

claudication pain in the leg after walking.

collaterals branches of smaller vessels.

Doppler pressure/levels measurement of the pressure in the blood vessels.

femoral, tibial, popliteal and profunda are all arteries.

haematoma localized internal collection of blood that sometimes occurs after injury or operation.

ischaemia deficiency in blood supply.

paraesthesia loss of sensation.

well perfused good supply of fluid (blood) through the blood vessels.

Example 11.4   Surgical summary – letter form (to GP)

Thank you for referring this 67-year-old man. He previously underwent **ERCP** with clearing of his common bile duct followed by **cholecystectomy** for **cholelithiasis** three years ago. He has remained very well since his surgery until four days ago when he developed **epigastric** pain following a meal. The pain was constant with no radiation. He vomited twice over 48 hours after which the pain resolved. The patient noticed pale stools and urine during this time but no **jaundice**.

On examination he looked well. There was a mild hint of **icteric sclera** but he was not overtly jaundiced. There was no evidence of anaemia and he was **apyrexial**. His chest was clinically clear and his abdomen was soft. He had no epigastric or right upper quadrant tenderness. His bowel sounds were normal and he had no evidence of abdominal masses or hepatomegaly. Rectal examination was normal. His left testicle was slightly **atrophic** compared to the right but this is a long-standing feature.

My impression is that he could have recurrent stones in the common bile duct and we need to exclude this. I have therefore requested urgent ultrasound examination. I feel we ought to exclude peptic ulcer and reflux oesophagitis and have requested gastroscopy. I have also requested full blood count, liver function tests, amylase, urine electrolytes and advised him to continue with a low-fat diet. I will review him next week.

Explanation of terms used in Example 11.4

apyrexial no pyrexia, (i.e. no fever).

atrophic wasting away, diminution in size.

cholecystectomy removal of the gall bladder.

cholelithiasis stones in the gall bladder.

epigastric an area at the top of the stomach in the midline (epigastrium).

ERCP endoscopic retrograde cholangiopancreatogram. This is a procedure for visualizing and removing stones in the common bile duct without major operation. (The common bile duct is referred to by initials, CBD.)

icteric sclera sclera of the eye affected with jaundice – yellow pigment. Jaundice can be caused by infection, or obstruction of the common bile duct by stones or tumour.

Example 11.5   Surgical summary – letter form (to GP)

Thank you for referring this 55-year-old-lady whom I saw in the clinic today. She is complaining of progressively worsening varicose veins in her left leg over the past years associated with **pruritis** and cramps in the leg. She has noticed oedema of her ankles in the hot weather. She has had previous **thrombophlebitis** 18 months ago but no history of deep vein thrombosis or ulceration. She is, I note, taking Prempak C for menopausal symptoms.

On examination she was rather obese with no evidence of anaemia or lymphadenopathy. There were no abnormal findings in her abdomen or any pelvic masses. She had no evidence of any saphenofemoral incompetence **bilaterally** or any extension of the long saphenous vein. She did have left lower leg varicosity with minor **venous flares** and some early **haemosiderin** pigmentation. She had some minor varicose veins in her left posterior calf but no evidence of short saphenous vein incompetence. Certainly her veins could be best treated with injection **sclerotherapy**. I have advised her to try and reduce weight and to wear support stockings. I have explained that injection sclerotherapy is contraindicated whilst she is on hormone replacement therapy. I have advised her to consult you with a view to stopping this before proceeding to sclerotherapy.

Explanation of terms used in Example 11.5

bilaterally   both sides.
haemosiderin pigmentation   skin discoloration caused by accumulation of haemoglobin derivative (also called haemosiderosis).
pruritis   itching.
sclerotherapy   injection of sclerosing solutions for the treatment of varicose veins or haemorrhoids.
thrombophlebitis   inflammation of a vein associated with a clot formation.
varicosity   a varicose vein condition – distended vein.
venous flares   area of redness associated with varicose veins.

Examples of ultrasound and X-ray reports

Example 11.6   Ultrasound of abdomen

The gall bladder is distended to approximately 10 cm in length, 6 cm in width and 3.5 cm in depth; it shows a thickened wall to a maximum wall thickness of approximately 0.8 cm and contains multiple bright echoes casting acoustic shadows characteristic of gallstones. The intrahepatic ducts were of normal calibre but the CBD (common bile duct) is dilated to a maximum of 0.9 cm diameter and contains a bright echo at its distal end showing a maximum length of 0.8 cm consistent with a calculus in the common bile duct. Liver, pancreas, spleen and kidneys, **NAD**. Small bilateral basal pleural effusions evident. $\rightarrow$

> The aorta was slightly **atheromatous** but showed normal calibre over its proximal 12 cm at maximum diameter of 2.1 cm.

Example 11.7   Ultrasound of abdomen

> Free fluid is present within the **peritoneal cavity**. The gall bladder is free of calculi. The gall bladder wall appears thickened – this is presumably oedematous secondary to **ascites**. The liver is of normal homogeneous echogenicity and the CBD does not appear dilated.
>
> Normal appearances of spleen, pancreas and both kidneys. The bladder was moderately distended. No evidence of intraluminal filling defect. **Prostatic** enlargement noted.

Example 11.8   Barium enema

> Barium passed freely around the caecum and refluxed into the terminal ileum. Apart from one or two scattered **diverticula** there was no evidence of any intrinsic or extrinsic bowel lesion. In particular, there was no evidence to suggest a pelvic mass lesion.

Example 11.9   Double-contrast barium enema

> There is some shortening of the large bowel in the region of the sigmoid, the appearances being consistent with a limited sigmoid resection with end-to-end anastomosis.
>
> Redundancy is noted in the upper descending colonic and splenic flexure.
>
> No abnormalities demonstrated at the anastomotic site or in the remaining large bowel. No evidence of polyps or recurrent tumour.

Example 11.10   Barium meal

> The swallowing mechanism was normal. No evidence of **hiatus hernia**.
>
> There was some reflux into the lower oesophagus. The gastric fundus and body were normal. The stomach was seen to contain rather thickened **rugae** consistent with hypersecretion. The flow of contrast into the duodenum was somewhat slow although the gastric antrum was normal.
>
> The duodenal cap was somewhat deformed presumably due to previous surgery.
>
> No evidence of active ulceration. The rest of the duodenum was normal.

Explanation of terms used in Examples 11.6–11.10

anastomosis surgical joining together of two pieces of bowel or blood vessel, to allow flow.

ascites abnormal accumulation of fluid in peritoneal cavity.

atheromatous the presence of fatty or lipid material, atheroma or plaque in blood vessels.

diverticula small blind pouches formed by bulging out of the lining through the wall of the colon.

hiatus hernia protrusion of abdominal content through the oesophageal hiatus of the diagphragm.

peritoneal cavity space within the peritoneum (intraperitoneal as opposed to extraperitoneal).

prostatic referring to the prostate gland.

rugae ridges or folds.

Example 11.11   Right femoral arteriogram (angiogram)

A right femoral approach was used and a size 7 **French** straight catheter was inserted. The lower aorta was normal and both common iliac vessels were within normal limits.

Right lower limb
The right external iliac artery was relatively smooth. The common femoral artery was smooth but the superficial artery was completely occluded at its origin. The profunda femoris was patent and numerous collaterals emanating from these vessels re-anastomosed to form an irregular popliteal artery. This was patent to the **trifurcation**. The anterior tibial artery terminated in the form of collaterals only a few cm distal to the origin. The **peroneal** artery was patent throughout and crossed the ankle at the dorsalis pedis. The posterior tibial artery was also patent throughout its length although irregular in the lower third. It did however cross the ankle to the foot.

Explanation of terms used in Example 11.11

French refers to size of a tube.

peroneal pertaining to the lateral aspect of the leg.

trifurcation site of separation into three branches (bifurcation two branches).

Example 11.12   Intravenous urogram (IVU)

Contrast medium administered intravenously.

Both kidneys are normal in size, shape and position. The right kidney measures 11 cm and the left kidney measures 12.3 cm. Both kidneys excreted contrast promptly and symmetrically. There are bilateral partial →

duplex systems with a dilated pelvicalyceal system of the lower **moiety** on the left and slight dilatation of the right mid-pole calyces. Both upper pole moieties are normal. There is no evidence of obstruction. The right-sided partial system unites on the level of the renal pelvis and the left unites at the same **PUJ** level. The bladder is normal and empties well on micturition. The post-micturition film infers left-sided reflux to the lower moiety. There is decreased cortex overlying the left moiety. Suggest **DTPA** scan to determine the relative function.

Explanation of terms used in Example 11.12

DTPA   a radionucleotide (see Chapter 7).
moiety   any equal part, half or portion.
PUJ   pelviureteric junction.

Other terms commonly occurring in kidney and bladder X-ray reports

Term	Meaning
cystitis	inflammation of the bladder.
cystitis cystica	a chronic form of cystitis.
hydronephrosis	distention of inside of kidney, by urine that can't flow past an obstruction.
parenchyma	tissue of an organ.
renal cortical scarring	scarring of the outer part of the kidney (cortex), probably due to infection.
trabeculation of bladder	formation of cords or crossbars in the bladder.
ureterocoele	prolapse of the tip of the ureter into the bladder.
vesicoureteric reflux	abnormal backflow of urine from bladder up the ureter. Several causes.

General surgical operations

Name	Procedure

Abdominal operations

appendicectomy	removal of appendix.
cholecystectomy	removal of gall bladder.
colostomy	a temporary or permanent opening of the bowel through the abdominal wall.
ERCP	endoscopic retrograde cholangiopancreatogram.
gastrectomy	removal of stomach.
hemicolectomy	removal of half the colon.
herniorrhaphy	repair of hernia.

Name	Procedure
laparotomy	exploratory abdominal operation.
oesophagectomy	removal of oesophagus.
sigmoid colectomy and review of colostomy reversal }	removal of sigmoid colon and possible closure of colostomy.
splenectomy	removal of spleen.
vagotomy	cutting the vagus nerve (may be done in cases of duodenal or gastric ulcer).

Blood vessel operations

abdominal aortic Dacron graft }	repair of abdominal aortic aneurysm.
CABS	coronary artery by-pass surgery.
femoral embolectomy	removal of embolus from femoral artery.
lumbar sympathectomy	excision of some portion of the sympathetic nervous system in the lumbar area.
femoropopliteal bypass graft	insertion of graft between the femoral and popliteal arteries.

There are many operations in bypass arterial surgery with anastomosis and grafting in cases of aneurysms and arteries narrowed by atheroma.

Common operations for varicose veins

saphenofemoral disconnection	saphenous vein is ligated at the groin where it joins the femoral vein.
stripping	a wire device called a stripper is threaded through the lumen of the vein from groin to ankle and the wire and vein then pulled from the groin.
Trendelenburg	is the name for the operation which is performed to remove weakened portions of veins and pockets in which thrombi (clots) might lodge. Stripping and saphenofemoral disconnection form part of the operation.

Genitourinary operations

circumcision	surgical removal of foreskin (prepuce).
cystoscopy	looking into bladder with the aid of a cystoscope.
nephrectomy	removal of a kidney.
orchidectomy	removal of a testicle.
re-implantation of ureter	Usually means repositioning ureter into bladder in cases of urinary problems and abnormalities.

Name	Procedure
repair vesicovaginal fistula	repair of bladder – vagina fistula.
TURP	transurethral resection of prostate.
TURBT	transurethral resection of bladder tumour.
vasectomy	male sterilization procedure.

Rectal operations

abdominal perineal excision of rectum often referred to as 'AP' resection	removal of rectum; performed in cases of cancer of rectum.
anal stretch	performed in some cases of haemorrhoids or stricture.
draining ischiorectal abscess	aseptic drainage and cleaning of abscess.
excision fissure *in ano*	repair of painful crack in skin of anus.
excision of pilonidal sinus	repair of sinus (recess) in the sacrococcygeal region.
haemorrhoidectomy	removal of haemorrhoids.
repair of fistula	repair of communication or passage which should not exist (e.g. between rectum and vagina).
sponge rectopexy	operation to correct rectal prolapse.

Other operations

lumpectomy	removal of a lump.
mastectomy	removal of a breast.
myotomy	cutting or dissection of muscular tissue.
polypectomy	removal of a polyp.
thyroglossal cyst excision	removal of cyst from throat and neck area.
thyroidectomy	removal of thyroid gland.

Part IV
Terminology for Specialities

Chapter 12
Orthopaedics and Rheumatology

Knowledge of the terminology relating to bones, joints and muscles as well as being familiar with their diseases is needed by the secretary working in orthopaedics, rheumatology and X-ray. This chapter also contains some orthopaedic and rheumatology reports, bone X-ray reports, examples of some orthopaedic operations, and the names of nails and screws used in orthopaedic procedures.

Terminology

Some terms	*Meaning*

Parts of bones

apophysis	outgrowth of bone such as a process.
condyle	rounded projection or ridge.
epicondyle	projection above an articulating surface.
epiphysis	end of long bones where growth occurs in childhood (adj. epiphyseal).
foramen	a hole perforating a bone for the passage of nerves and blood vessels.
fossa	depression in a bone.
lamina or lamella	thin plate of bone.
meatus or canal	a bony tunnel.
metaphysis	a wider part of the extremity of long bones.
notch	indentation in a bone.
periosteum	fibrous membrane covering bone.
process	projection from a bone.
shaft	long slender part of long bones.
spine	short pointed eminence.
tubercle	a smaller process.
tuberosity or trochanter	a broad rough surface.

Conditions affecting bones

avascular necrosis	death of bone due to poor blood supply
callus formation	occurs after fractures as part of the healing process.

Some terms	Meaning
degenerative changes	due to ageing and arthritis.
erosive changes	seen in rheumatoid arthritis.
exostosis	excess bony formation often associated with arthritis.
dimineralization	excessive elimination of mineral or organic salts.
fractures	some common ones:
	avulsion
	blow out
	Colles' (wrist)
	comminuted
	compression
	flake
	greenstick
	Pott's (ankle)
	spiral
	subcapital
	transcervical.
hyperostosis	excessive growth of bone.
loss of articular surface	loss of joint surface.
metastatic changes	secondary deposits in bone.
neoplastic changes	change caused by tumour.
osteoarthritis	degeneration of a joint.
osteophyte	bony outgrowths adjacent to osteoarthritic joint.
osteoporosis	loss of density in bones.
porotic bones	bones that are less dense when seen on the X-ray.

Other useful terms

genu	knee.
hallux	great toe.
metatarsus	part of foot between tarsus and the toes.
osteochondritis	disease of growth or ossification centre in children known by various names according to bone involved.
Paget's disease	disease of the bones causing deformity (osteitis deformans).
pes	foot.
plantar	pertaining to the sole of the foot.
slipped epiphysis	dislocation of epiphysis of a bone commonly the femur.
stippled epiphysis	chondrodystrophia calcifans.
talipes	clubfoot, also referred to as congenital talipes equinovarus (CTEV).

Some terms	*Meaning*
torticollis	wryneck, a contracted state of the cervical muscles.

Conditions of the spine

ankylosing spondylitis	a disease characterized by immobility and consolidation (ankylosis) of joints and inflammation of the vertebrae (spondylitis).
coccydynia	pain from the coccyx.
dysraphism	incomplete closure of primary neural tube in the spinal cord.
kyphosis	hump back.
lordosis	anterior concavity in the curvature of the spine.
prolapsed intervertebral disc	PID; slipped disc.
sciatica	pain along the course of the sciatic nerve.
scoliosis	sideways curvature of the spine.
spina bifida	congenital gap in the posterior part of the bony arch of the spine.
spina bifida occulta	concealed gap of no significance normally and only seen on the X-ray.

Conditions of the knee

anterior cruciate ligament tear	important ligament in the knee joint sometimes torn in injuries to the knee.
chondromalacia patellae	softening of the cartilage of the knee cap (patella) causing pain behind the knee(s).
genu recurvatum	hyper-extension of the knee.
genu valgum	knock knees.
genu varum	bow leg.
medial meniscus injuries	damage to the medial semilunar cartilage in the knee joint.
osteochondritis dissecans	condition whereby an area of bone with its overlying cartilage gradually separates and may form a loose body within the joint.
pre-patellar bursitis	inflammation of the bursa (sac like cavity) in front of the knee cap.
rupture of quadriceps muscles	rupture of the four muscles in the thigh which extend the knee.

Conditions of the foot

Achilles tendon injuries	rupture of the strong tendon at the back of the heel.
hallux malleus	hammer toe.
hallux rigidus	painful stiffening of great toe.
hallux valgus	angulation of great toe towards other toes causing bunions.

Some terms	Meaning
hallux varus	angulation of great toe away from other toes.
metatarsalgia	pain in metatarsal region.
Morton's neuroma	a swollen nerve under the foot that is painful.
pes planus/valgus	flat foot.
pes pronatus/supinatus	deformed foot.
plantar fasciitis	inflammation of the band of fibrous tissue on the sole of the foot.
talipes	club foot.

Conditions of the hand and wrist

carpal tunnel syndrome	trapped nerve in the wrist.
de Quervain's disease	painful tenosynovitis due to narrowness of the common tendon sheath of the tendons serving the thumb.
Dupuytren's contracture	flexion deformity of a finger due to thickening and fibrosis of the fascia of palm.
Heberden's nodes	swelling around the distal interphalangeal joints of the fingers; associated with generalized osteoarthritis.
tenosynovitis	inflammation of tendon sheath.
Volkmann's contracture	contracture usually involving fingers or wrist after severe injury.

Conditions of shoulder and elbow

frozen shoulder	disability of the shoulder joint.
golfer's elbow	disability due to medial epicondylitis.
tennis elbow	disability due to inflammation of the extensor tendon attachment to the lateral humeral condyle.

Muscles

It is useful to know the names of some muscles for orthopaedics and rheumatology but a comprehensive medical dictionary should provide you with information about unfamiliar ones. Some muscles are named according to their function, so there are abductors, adductors, extensors, flexors, supinators and pronators. Some are described as longus, brevis (short) magnus, maximus and minimi.

Some shoulder and arm muscles

biceps
brachialis
deltoid
flexor or extensor carpi radialis   FCR or ECRL (longus) and ECRB (brevis)
flexor or extensor carpi ulnaris   FCU, ECU

infraspinatus
subscapularis
supraspinatus
teres major or minor

Some hip and thigh muscles

gluteal   there are three: gluteus maximus, medius and minimus
hamstring
quadriceps   include vastus lateralis, medialis, and intermedius
psoas; there are three: brevis, longus and tertius

Some leg muscles

flexor longus hallucis (FHL)
gastrocnemius
peroneal

Muscles containing

digitorum	refer to	fingers and toes
pollicis		thumb
hallucis		great toe
palmaris		hand
plantaris		foot

interosseous muscles are in the hand and foot.

Examples of orthopaedic summaries with explanations of terms used

Example 12.1   Orthopaedic summary

Diagnosis

Prolapsed intervertebral disc L4/5

Operation

Laminectomy of right L4/5

History

This 42-year-old gentleman was admitted complaining of back and right leg pain. He had paraesthesia in his right toes and the sole of his foot.

Examination

Straight-leg raising on the right was reduced to 25° with pain down the right leg. There was weakness of the right ankle dorsiflexion and extension.   →

Sensation was decreased on the right side over the L5/S1 region. Reflexes were intact. A **lumbar radiculogram** was performed on the day after admission which showed a large central and right sided disc prolapse at the L4/L5 level

Operation

Right laminectomy. Large disc found which was removed with difficulty due to the presence of adhesions. At the end of the procedure the L5 root lay free.

Postoperatively the patient made a good recovery and was discharged two weeks later.

Explanation of terms used in Example 12.1

laminectomy   excision of posterior arch of a vertebra performed to gain access to a prolapsed intervertebral disc.

lumbar radiculogram   X-ray of spine/spinal cord using contrast-medium; also for examining lumbar nerve roots.

Example 12.2   Orthopaedic summary

Diagnosis

Garden III transcervical fracture left neck of femur

Operation

Cemented left Thompson's hemiarthroplasty

History

This 90-year-old patient was admitted following a fall in which he hurt his left leg.

Examination

The left leg was externally rotated with minimal shortening. There was pain on all movements of his left hip. X-rays revealed a Garden III transcervical fracture of the left neck of the femur.

Operation

Cemented left Thompson's hemiarthroplasty.

Postoperative check X-rays showed a good position and the patient was discharged back to the nursing home where he was resident.

Example 12.3   Orthopaedic summary

Diagnosis

>Dislocated 4th and 5th metacarpals of right hand at metacarpo–hamate joint with flake fracture proximal 5th metacarpal.

Operation

>Manipulation under anaesthetic (MUA) of right hand.

History

This 26-year-old man was admitted following an injury to the right hand when he punched a brick wall. He had been drinking alcohol all day.

Examination

The right hand was bruised and very tender. Sensation and pulses were intact. X-rays revealed dislocated 4th and 5th metacarpals right hand.

Operation

Manipulation under GA [general anaesthetic] right hand.

The patient made an uneventful recovery and was discharged in a plaster of Paris.

Bone X-rays summaries

Example 12.4   X-ray report – left tibia and fibula

A 'K' nail has been inserted through the length of the tibia across the fractured mid-shaft. This fracture has now healed with abundant callus formation. The two fractures in the mid-shaft of the fibula have healed. Condition and position as shown

The screw running in the AP [anteroposterior] projection is seen to be protruding through the skin surface.

Example 12.5   X-ray report – left tibia

A flake is noted off the medial side of the lower portion of the tibia. A healed fracture of the upper shaft of the fibula is noted.

No evidence of osteomylitis [infection of the bone] is seen associated with the plate or screws. There is no displacement of the plate.

Example 12.6   X-ray report – right foot

> There is no evidence of gouty erosions. Slight soft-tissue swelling is seen over the medial portion of the 1st MTP joint [metatarsophalangeal joint]. No other abnormality is seen.

Example 12.7   X-ray report – left knee standing

> The knee shows a degree of valgus deformity [lower leg angled outwards].
>
> Degenerative changes with narrowing of both compartments of the knee joint, spiking of the tibial spines, osteophyte formation medially, laterally and at the patellofemoral joint is noted.

Example 12.8   X-ray report – left shoulder

> No abnormality is seen in the left shoulder joint. Early degenerative changes are present in the left acromioclavicular joint. There is no evidence of any abnormal soft-tissue calcification in the left shoulder region.

Example 12.9   X-ray report – left hand

> There is a small flake fracture from the proximal articular surface of the middle phalanx of the index finger seen on the oblique view only.

Example 12.10   X-ray report – right elbow

> No evidence of recent bony injury seen. Some degenerative changes are seen, and some calcification is seen over the lateral aspects of the epicondyles. This may either be in bursa, or in tendon.

Example 12.11   X-ray report – pelvis and left hip

> Marked degenerative changes seen in the left hip joint where there is complete loss of joint space, and distortion of the femoral head likely to be related to avascular necrosis. The femoral head is migrating upwards and the acetabular roof is also expanded upwards. On the right, the hip joint appears relatively normal. However, there is a possible abnormal angulation of the femoral neck on the femoral shaft. The patient is rotated on this film, but the appearances are suggestive of an intertrochanteric fracture of the left hip. A lateral view of the left hip is suggested to confirm or exclude a fracture.

Example 12.12   X-ray report – cervical spine

> Moderate degenerative changes are seen in the mid-lower cervical region with slight disc space narrowing at C5/6 level, and some anterior osteophyte formation at C4/5, 5/6 and 6/7 levels. The neural canal is of normal dimensions and is uncompromised.
>
> Bilateral cervical ribs [supernumerary ribs arising from cervical vertebra] are noted.

Example 12.13   X-ray report – lumbar spine

> There is a spondylolisthesis of L4 on L5.
>
> The forward slip of L4 on L5, however is not significantly changed since the previous film. No defect in the pars interarticularis is seen on the oblique view. Degenerative changes are demonstrated in the posterior joints of L4/5 and L5/S1 and small osteophytes are also seen at L3/4.

Some orthopaedic operations

Back

decompression spinal fusion
discectomy
fenestration
laminectomy
microdiscectomy
spinal fusion.

Hip

dynamic hip screw
Thompson's hemiarthroplasty
total hip replacement (THR).

Knee

arthroscopy (also performed on elbow or shoulder)
Jones' procedure right knee (repair of ligament)
meniscectomy
patellectomy
tibial osteotomy.

Foot

correction hammer toes
Helal arthroplasty (artificial joint big toe)

operations for hallux valgus   bunionectomy
Keller's arthroplasty
metatarsal osteotomy

Leg and ankle

internal fixation medial malleolus
release of hamstrings (hamstring tenotomy)
removal 'K' nail from tibia
tibial osteotomy.

Hand and wrist

arthrodesis wrist, excision ulnar styloid
carpal tunnel release/decompression
de Quervains
Dupuytren's contracture.

Other procedures

A O plate and bone graft
excision of ganglion
excision olecranon bursa elbow
fasciectomy
manipulation under anaesthetic (MUA).

Some plates, nails and screws commonly used

A O plating, AO nail
Charnley clamp
Denham pin
Dynamic Condylar plate (DCP)
Dynamic hip screw (DHS)
gamma interlocking nail
Grosse-Kempf nail (G-K nail)
Herbert screws
Kirschner wire ('K'-wire)
Kuntscher ('K' nail) intramedullary nail
Roehampton external fixator
Smith-Petersen nail
Steinmann pin.

Conditions treated by the rheumatologist

Arthritis

Many different types such as:
acute arthritis

Charcot's arthritis
chronic villous (form of rheumatoid) arthritis
Marie-Strumpell arthritis
neuropathic arthritis
osteoarthritis
palindromic arthritis/rheumatism
polyarthritis
polymyalgia rheumatica
psoriatic arthritis
rheumatoid arthritis – seropositive and seronegative
septic arthritis
Still's disease (juvenile chronic arthritis).

Some rheumatology terms

gout   excess uric acid in the blood. Crystals of urate can accumulate in joints causing pain.

rheumatism   a lay term referring to musculoskeletal pain.

SLE   systemic lupus erythematosus. An autoimmune generalized connective tissue disorder with skin eruption, arthralgia and other symptoms.

Example of rheumatology summary with explanation of terms used

Example 12.14   Rheumatology report

Diagnosis

Seronegative rheumatoid arthritis

History

This patient developed problems with joint pains 9 months previously following an attack of mumps. She was particularly troubled by a swollen, tender, painful and relatively immobile left knee. However, she was also affected in the right wrist, neck, right knee and first metatarsophalangeal joint.

Examination

There was essentially no abnormality except in the joints. The left knee in particular was slightly inflamed, hot to the touch with a small **effusion**. Flexion was limited to 60°.

Management

The patient was admitted for **arthroscopy** and synovial biopsy to confirm the diagnosis. The left knee fluid was aspirated and sent for culture and   →

sensitivity. Hypertrophic **synovial villi** were noted around the patellar edge. The medial patellar **facet** was irregular. Both femoral condyles were intact. The **medial meniscus** had an irregular free edge. The **anterior cruciate ligament** was intact. Synovial biopsies were taken.

Results

Histology: **synovium** was heavily infiltrated by plasma cells with some aggregates of lymphocytes. No **fibrinoid necrosis** was seen. Appearances were suggestive of rheumatoid arthritis.

X-ray: Affected joints showed no erosive changes. Early degenerative changes were seen.

Bone scan: confirmed diagnosis.

Intravenous urogram (IVU): within normal limits.

Full blood count: nad.

RA latex tests: RA HA: negative.

Autoantibodies: negative.

Bacteriology including acid fast bacilli on synovial fluid: negative.

Future management

Drugs on discharge
   flurbiprofen   100 mg bd.

The patient will be seen in the outpatient clinic and these results will be discussed with her. She will then probably be started on second line antirheumatoid agents.

Explanation of terms used in Example 12.14

anterior cruciate ligament   important ligament in the knee.
arthroscopy   looking into a joint with an arthroscope, normally the knee.
effusion   presence of fluid in a space, such as a joint or lining of the lungs.
facet   plane surface usually on a bone.
fibrinoid   resembling fibrin.
flurbiprofen   a non-steroidal antiinflammatory drug (NSAID).
medial and lateral meniscii   crescent-shaped structures in the knee joint.
necrosis   death of tissue.
synovial membrane   this lines the cavity of joints and secretes a fluid (synovial fluid).
synovial villi   small projections of the synovial membranes into the joint cavity.
synovium   synovial membrane.

Chapter 13
Dermatology

This chapter focuses on skin conditions, and includes sample summaries as well as a comprehensive glossary of disease conditions and terms.

For basic anatomy of the skin, the reader is referred to Chapter 5.

This chapter may also be of use to the secretary in the Histology department as there is an overlap in the terms used by both histologists and dermatologists to describe various tissues, cells and skin appearances.

Examples of dermatology summaries with explanations of terms used

Example 13.1   Dermatology summary – letter form

Thank you for referring this patient. I entirely agree that the skin eruption is unlikely to be due to a drug reaction to either his long term Zyloric [drug given for gout] or his recently introduced Indocid [drug given for pain in gout, rheumatic and musculo-skeletal conditions].

I agree that he is a **psoriatic** with plaque lesions on his knees and lateral calves. However, there are vague pink less scaly lesions on his wrists, abdomen and thighs which need explaining. Perhaps this is the beginning of a **guttate psoriasis** associated with his toe **arthropathy**, but I am sure we should check an **ASO titre**, throat swab and **Australia antigen**. Meanwhile, for treatment I have suggested penicillin V 500 mg qid for six days against the possibility that there is a streptococcus in his body (there was no lymphadenopathy nor throat infection today). For the psoriasis I have suggested Polytar bars and 5% coal tar solution in Eumovate ointment twice daily.

Explanation of terms used in Example 13.1

anthropathy   disease of a joint.

ASO titre   antistreptolysin-O titre – a blood test done to check if recent streptococcal infection has occurred.

Australia antigen (HBsAg)   positive in patients who have or are carriers for virus causing serum hepatitis B. *Extremely* infective.

guttate psoriasis form of psoriasis in which the lesions are small and may begin after sunburn or streptococcal infection.

psoriatic one who suffers from psoriasis.

Example 13.2 Dermatology summary – letter form

> Thank you for referring this 37-year-old lady with a violent eruption of **acne vulgaris** on her face. There are **comedones**, pustules, cysts and scars. Surprisingly she had no lesions in her teens and indeed her face was clear until last year. She then had a violent eruption on her neck spreading to her face which was so bad that she came up to Casualty. She has had oxytetracyline and flucloxacillin with some benefit.
>
> I feel that the violence of this eruption means that there must be some systemic factor at play. She is married and has two children of 8 and 11 and has been taking Microgynon [oral contraceptive] for three years now and has a normal menstrual cycle. She eats much in the way of fish and took cod liver oil capsules, two nightly for twelve months until nine months ago. She does not take large quantities of fizzy drinks. Over the past two years she has used simple cleansing products and a facial dry skin lotion.
>
> On general examination she had a slightly puffy face with **hirsute** upper lip. This may be familial but I did wonder about early **Cushing's**. Secondary sexual characteristics were normal. She had violent acne to her cheeks today.
>
> I have taken a swab from a broken pustule and have decided to investigate her **FBC**, testosterone level, cortisol level and pelvic ultrasound.
>
> For treatment I have recommended clindamycin capsules 1 bd and clindamycin lotion daily.
>
> I will see her again in three weeks' time.

Explanation of terms used in Example 13.2

comedones 'blackheads'.

Cushing's syndrome an endocrine disease due to neoplasm of the adrenal cortex or anterior lobe of the pituitary. Characterized by 'moon' face and extra facial hair.

FBC full blood count.

hirsute hairy.

Example 13.3 Dermatology summary – letter form

> Thank you for asking me to see this 12-month-old child with some eight yellow papules scattered over his body. The first one appeared on his scalp at the age of one month and the others have gradually grown, perhaps those on his scalp are already flattening. There were lesions on his scrotum, behind the right ear, four on the scalp and one on the left flank. There was a
>
> →

tiny lesion developing on the left side of his chin. These are naevoxantho-endotheliomata, benign collections of lipid laden **macrophages**. This is a rare condition.

I have never seen such lesions associated with **hyperlipidaemia** but in the context of this child's grandfather having hyperlipidaemia I thought it wisest to have the child checked in the same laboratory. He also has two **café-au-lait** patches on his abdomen and there is an occasional association between juvenile **xanthogranulomata** and **neurofibromatosis**. It may be worth while biopsying one of these juvenile xanthogranulomata to have histological confirmation.

Explanation of terms used in Example 13.3

café-au-lait   pigmented macules of light brown colour.

hyperlipidaemia   excess of lipids (lipids = fats) in the blood which can lead to heart disease

juvenile xanthogranuloma   a dermatosis beginning in childhood consisting of yellow papules or nodules. Also called naevoxantho-endothelioma.

macrophages   phagocytic cells, part of the reticuloendothelial system.

neurofibromatosis   a familial condition marked by changes in the nervous system, muscles and bones and skin due to formation of multiple soft tumours.

xanthoma   a yellowish papule, nodule or plaque in the skin due to fatty deposits.

Example 13.4   Dermatology summary – letter form

Thank you so much for asking me to see this little boy and for your helpful letter about him. As you say, it may well be that this child with **IgA deficiency** is complicating the issue of his constitutional **atopic dermatitis**.

On examination today however this was a perfectly standard atopic dermatitis; his brother has continuing low-grade eczema. I am sure his retardation is a factor in his continual scratching and rubbing of his hands and the perpetuation of the eczema at this site. There has been considerable improvement since your prescription.

I made the following points to mother today:

1.   Diet   I am generally unenthusiastic about the beneficial effects of dairy product-free regimens beneficially influencing eczema.

2.   **Antihistamines**   I agree with you that a sedative antihistamine is often very helpful especially when used at night. Mother found Triludan 1–2 tablets twice daily very helpful. I have suggested that she might try Vallergan at night.

→

> 3. Local treatment   I have made minor refinements to the regimen:
>
> Balneum to be added to baths rather than Alpha Keri; aqueous cream to be used as a soap substitute on the hands; 1% hydrocortisone cream to be applied to the raw and red areas at night before the emollient zinc and castor oil cream one part, oily cream BP nine parts. **Calaband** bandages overnight when necessary.

Explanation of terms used in Example 13.4

antihistamines   group of drugs used to counteract effect of histamine release in sensitivity reactions.

atopic dermatitis   skin inflammation (dermatitis) due to allergy.

Calaband bandages   zinc paste and calamine bandage.

***IgA* deficiency**   an immunoglobin deficiency affecting antibody reaction and immunity.

Glossary of other dermatological and related terms

Term	Meaning
acanthosis	thickening of the prickle cell layer of the skin.
acanthosis nigricans	diffuse acanthosis with grey, brown or black pigmentation.
achromasia	lack of normal pigment in the skin.
acne	inflammatory papulopustular skin condition. Many types: atrophica conglobata erythematosa keratosa vulgaris.
acneiform	resembling acne.
acrochordon	soft pendulous growths occurring on neck, eyelids and axilla.
actinic	producing chemical action, said of certain rays of light.
allergen	substance capable of producing allergy.
alopecia	baldness. May be: *adnata* congenital *areata* inflammatory, usually reversible type *cicatrisata/orbularis* irreversible *pityrodes* associated with dandruff.
angiokeratoma/ angiokeratosis	warty growth in groups.

Term	Meaning
angiolipoma	benign blood vessel tumour (angioma) containing fatty tissue.
angioneurotic oedema	painless temporary swellings of the subcutaneous tissues usually of the face, may be due to allergy or emotional factors.
antihistamine	a drug used to counteract the effects of allergy, particularly in cases of hay fever and allergic rashes.
antimetabolite	substance which interferes with the utilization of an essential metabolite produced during metabolism.
apocrine	type of glandular secretion.
aqueous cream	water-based cream used in dermatological treatments.
atopy	clinical hypersensitive state or allergy with hereditary predisposition.
atrophia unguium	atrophy of the nails.
atrophia cutis senilis	senile atrophy of the skin.
bacterid	skin eruption caused by bacterial infection.
basal cell carcinoma (BCC)	form of skin cancer.
bulla (pl. bullae)	a blister or elevated lesion of the skin (adj. bullate, bullous).
callosity	a callus.
callous	nature of callus, hard.
callus	localized hyperplasia of horny layer of epidermis *or* network of woven bone as healing process in fractures.
cellulitis	local skin infection usually due to the bacterium streptococcus.
cheilitis	inflammation affecting the lips.
cheiropompholyx	intensely itchy skin eruption on the side of digits, palm and soles.
chloasma	hyperpigmentation in circumscribed areas of the skin.
chondrodermatitis	inflammatory process involving cartilage and skin.
cicatrix	scar.
collodian	highly flammable syrupy liquid which dries to clear film, used as protection to skin to close small cuts or to hold dressings in place.
colloid	glue-like, gelatinous substance from colloid degeneration.
comedo	'blackhead'.

Term	*Meaning*
corium	true skin or dermis.
cryotherapy	therapeutic use of cold.
cysts	many forms – epithelial, sebaceous/epidermal.

dermatitis	skin inflammation. Many forms:
	    actinic (due to sunlight)
	    allergic
	    contact
	    eczematous.

dermatofibroma	a fibrous tumour-like nodule of the skin.
dermatomycosis	a superficial fungal infection of the skin.
dermatomyositis	a collagen disease that is a serious disease involving connective tissue.
dermatophyte	a fungus parasitic upon the skin.
desloughing	getting rid of dead tissue (slough). Used to cleanse wounds or lesions to avoid/minimize infection.
desquamation	shedding of the epithelial elements, chiefly of the skin, in scales or sheets.
dhobie's itch	allergic contact dermatitis caused originally by marking fluid in Indian laundry, term now used for ringworm of the groin.
discoid	disc shaped.
dyschromia	any disorder of pigmentation of the hair or skin.
dyshidrosis	pruritic skin eruption on digits, palms, or soles of feet.
dyskeratosis	abnormal or premature keratinization of the keratinocytes, cells in the epidermis.
ecthyma	a shallowly eruptive form of impetigo.
eczema	a form of dermatitis.
emollient	an agent that softens or soothes the skin.
emulsions	used in dermatology as lubricants and ointments.
erysipelas	contagious disease of the skin due to Group A haemolytic streptococci.
erysipeloid	infective dermatitis or cellulitis due to infection with *Erysipelothrix insidiosa*.
erythema multiforme	reddening of the skin; many forms; may be allergic.
erythema nodosum	inflammatory skin disease caused by general infection, characterized by painful red nodules on the shins.
erythrasma	bacterial infection of the folds of the skin.
erythrocyanosis	coarsely mottled bluish or red discoloration of legs and thighs, especially in girls.

Term	Meaning
erythroderma	abnormal redness of the skin over widespread areas of the body.
excoriation	results of scratching.
exfoliation	falling off of scales or layers (adj. exfoliative).
follicular	pertaining to a follicle.
folliculitis	infection of the hair follicles.
Fox-Fordyce disease	condition characterized by plugging of the pores of the sweat glands and vesiculation of the epidermis.
fungal hyphae	filaments of a fungus.
furunculosis	persistent recurrence or simultaneous occurrence of furuncles (boils).
gentian violet	an antibacterial, antifungal and antihelminthic (helminth – worm) dye used topically for infections of the skin.
giant urticaria	also called angioneurotic oedema.
glomus	small body mainly composed of fine arterioles.
Goeckerman's routine	therapy for treating psoriasis.
granuloma annulare	tumour-like mass of granulation tissue forming a ring.
haemangioma	an innocent tumour composed of dilated blood vessels, usually birthmarks. Cavernous haemangioma is a spongy swelling with large vascular spaces.
halo	luminous circle, word used to describe the appearance of some lesions.
herpes simplex	a viral infection which gives rise to localized vesicles in the skin and mucous membranes.
herpes zoster	'shingles'.
herpetic	pertaining to the nature of herpes.
hidradenitis suppurativa	inflammation of an apocrine sweat gland.
hirsute	hairy.
histiocytome	tumour containing histiocytes or macrophages, large debris-eating (phagocytic) cells of the reticuloendothelial system.
hydrops	abnormal accumulation of fluid in tissue or body cavity (dropsy).
hydropic	affected with dropsy.
hyperhidrosis	excessive perspiration.
hyperkeratosis	hypertrophy of the horny layer of the skin.
hyperplasia	abnormal increase in tissue volume by growth of new normal cells.
hypertrichosis	excessive hairiness, hirsutism.
hyposensitization	desensitization.

Term	Meaning
ichthyosis	any of several generalized skin disorders marked by dryness, roughness and scaliness.
impetigo	infection of the skin.
inspissated	being thickened, dried or made less fluid by evaporation.
intertrigo	superficial dermatitis in skin creases such as neck, groin or axilla.
Kaposi's sarcoma	malignant disease chiefly involving the skin, now seen in some patients with AIDS.
keloid	protuberant, prominent scar due to excessive collagen formation.
keratin	principal constituent of epidermis, hair, nails and horny tissues.
keratosis	horny wart-like growths. Many forms: pilar, seborrhoeic, solar.
keratocanthoma	benign papular lesion usually on the face.
keratoderma	hypertrophy of the horny layer of the skin.
keratolytic	promoting keratolysis which is loosening or separation of the horny layer of the skin.
koilonychia	mis-shapen nails.
kraurosis	dried, shrivelled condition.
kraurosis vulvae	atrophy of female external genitalia with intense itching and leukoplakic patches on the mucosa.
lentigo	flat brownish pigmented spot on the skin; 'deep' freckle.
lentigo maligna	malignant lentigo.
leukoderma	white areas of skin due to depigmentation.
leukoplakia	disease of the mucous membrane forming white thickened patches.
lichen	type of papular skin disease. Many varieties: amyloidosus chronicus simplex fribromucinoidosus (myxoedematous) nitidus pilaris planopilaris planus ruber moniliformis ruber planus sclerosus et atrophicus scrofulosorum (scrofulsus) simplex chronicus

Term	Meaning
	spinulosus
	striatus
	urticatus.
lichenification	thickening and hardening of the skin with exaggeration of its normal markings; can be caused by scratching.
lichenoid	resembling lichen.
livedo	discoloured patches on the skin (adj. livedoid).
lupus	these are two distinct conditions:

	lupus vulgaris	tuberculosis of the skin
	lupus erythematosis	discoid.
		systemic – systemic lupus erythematosis (SLE).

Term	Meaning
lymphangioma	tumour composed of new lymph spaces and channels.
macule	discoloured spot on the skin not raised above surface.
mastocytoma	a benign aggregation of mast cells forming a nodular tumour.
melanocyte	type of cell in the epidermis (adj. melanocytic).
melanoderma	abnormal increase in melanin in the skin with production of hyperpigmented patches.
melanoma	tumour of melanin pigmented cells. Malignant melanoma is a malignant skin tumour with a marked tendency to metastases.
melasma	dark pigmentation of the skin.
miliaria	cutaneous changes associated with retention of sweat, prickly heat.
milium	'whitehead'.
mitoses	ordinary process of cell division (adj. mitotic).
molluscum contagiosum	viral disease of the skin.
moniliasis	candidiasis, fungal infection with candida; 'thrush'.
mycosis fungoides	rare chronic malignant lymphoreticular neoplasm of the skin.
naevus(i)	general term for mole or haemangioma. Types:
	compound
	epithelial
	intradermal
	junctional
	pigmented.
necrobiosis	the physiological death of cells.

Term	*Meaning*
necrolysis	separation or exfoliation of necrotic tissue.
nummular	coin-shaped.
onychauxis	hypertrophy of nail.
onychogryphosis	deformed overgrowth of nail.
onycholysis	separation of all or part of the nail.
onychomycosis	fungal disease of the nails.
onychophagia	nail biting.
onychorrhexis	breaking or splitting of nails.
onychosis	disease of the nails.
papilloma	benign tumour derived from epithelium.
papule	a small circumscribed, solid, elevated lesion of the skin (adj. papular).
paronychia	inflammation involving the folds of tissue surrounding the fingernail.
pediculous	infested with lice.
pellagra	a syndrome caused by vitamin B deficient diet. Mental and digestive disturbances as well as skin signs such as cracks and sores around mouth, red scaly skin on neck and chest areas.
perilesional	located or occurring around a lesion.
photodermatitis	an abnormal state of skin in which light is an important causative factor.
photosensitization	abnormally heightened reactivity of the skin to sunlight.
pilomatrixoma	a benign calcifying epithelial neoplasm derived from hair and matrix cells.
pilosebaceous	pertaining to hair follicle and sebaceous gland.
pityriasis	a group of skin diseases with fine branny scales. May be: alba rosea rubra pilaris.
plaque	any patch or flat area.
poikiloderma	a condition characterized by pigmentary and atrophic changes giving a mottled appearance.
pompholyx	an intensely pruritic skin eruption on the sides of digits, palms or soles.
prurigo	an itchy skin eruption, dome-shaped with transient vesicle on top. May be: mitis nodularis simplex.
pruritis	itching (adj. pruritic).
psoriasis	chronic recurrent skin disease marked by bright red patches and silvery scales.

Term	Meaning
PUVA	photochemotherapy using Psoralens and UVA (long wave ultraviolet light).
reticular	having a net-like pattern or structure.
rhinophyma	a form of rosacea marked by redness, hyperplasia, swelling and congestion of the skin of the nose.
rhomboid	shaped like a rectangle skewed to one side so that the angles are oblique.
rosacea	chronic disease affecting skin of nose, forehead and cheeks (formerly called acne rosacea).
salicylic acid	used as a keratolytic.
sarcoidosis of skin	progressive generalized granulomatous reticulosis.
scabies	an infectious skin disease caused by the itch mite.
scleroderma	chronic hardening and shrinking of connective tissue.
seborrhoea	excessive discharge from the sebaceous glands.
seborrhoeic	affected with or of the nature of seborrhoea.
stellate	star-shaped.
striae atrophicae	atrophic, pinkish or purplish scar-like lesions later becoming silvery-white due to weakening of elastic tissues associated with pregnancy or obesity.
sycosis barbae	'barber's itch'. A condition affecting follicles of the beard.
syringocystadenoma	adenoma of the sweat glands.
syringoma	adenoma of the sweat glands.
systemic lupus erythematosis (SLE)	an autoimmune connective tissue disease. It can affect the skin or any organ in the body.
telangiectasia	a vascular lesion formed by dilation of a group of small blood vessels.
tinea	name applied to many different kinds of superficial fungal infections.
tinea pedis	'athlete's foot'.
ulcer	arteriosclerotic, trophic, stasis of leg, aphthous (mouth).
unguentum	ointment.
unguis	a fingernail or toenail.
urticaria	condition characterized by severe itching and weals. May be called 'hives' or 'nettle' rash',

Term	Meaning
	Caused by certain foods, stress or infection. Many different types.
UVA	long wave ultraviolet light (wavelength 320–400 nm).
UVB	short wave ultraviolet light (wavelength 290–320 nm).
vellus	the coat of fine hairs covering the body from childhood to puberty.
verruca	wart.
vesicle	small blister.
vesicular	made up of vesicles on the skin.
vitiligo	patches of depigmentation on the skin.
weal	raised stripe on the skin as caused by the lash of a whip; typical of urticaria. (May be spelt wheal.)
xanthelasma	condition affecting the eyelids characterized by yellow spots.
xanthogranuloma	tumour of fat (lipid)-laden macrophages.
xanthoma	a papule, nodule or plaque in the skin due to lipid deposits.
xeroderma	excessive dryness of the skin, mild form of ichthyosis.

Chapter 14
Ear, Nose and Throat

The ear, nose and throat (ENT) surgeon is concerned with conditions and diseases of the ear, nose, paranasal sinuses and throat. A brief anatomy is given in Chapter 5 together with details of the bones of the skull, and upper respiratory tract which you will find helpful if working in the department.

This chapter includes samples of skull X-rays and ENT letters together with lists of useful terms and ENT operations.

Examples of ENT summaries with explanations of terms used

Ear, nose and throat (ENT) patients are frequently sent for skull X-rays, usually to detect infection of the sinuses. Below are two skull X-ray reports but in these cases both patients have had X-rays because of injury.

Example 14.1   ENT skull X-ray report

> No abnormality seen in the skull vault.
>
> The **sella** is within normal limits.
>
> The **pineal** is calcified.
>
> There is no evidence of displacement in the midline structures.
>
> The sinuses are clear.

Explanation of terms used in Example 14.1

pineal   gland or body in the cerebrum (see Endocrine System, Chapter 5).
sella   sella turcica, a depression on the upper surface of the sphenoid bone.

Example 14.2   Tomograms of right orbit

> There is a fracture through the inferior orbital floor extending for approximately 1.0–1.5 cm posteriorly into the **orbit**. It is involving the inferior orbital canal.   →

> Associated soft-tissue swelling is seen in the superior aspect of the right maxillary **antrum** associated with this blow-out fracture. A second blow-out fracture is seen in the postero-superior aspect of the orbital wall as seen on cuts 5.0 and 5.5 cm.
>
> A fracture of the nasal bones is present.

Explanation of terms used in Example 14.2

antrum cavity or sinus. Maxillary sinus is called the antrum of Highmore.

orbit bony cavity containing the eyeball, its muscles, nerves and vessels. The ethmoid, frontal, lacrimal, nasal, palatine, sphenoid and zygomatic bones and maxilla contribute to its bony walls.

tomogram form of X-ray examination which can produce images in the form of slices of a single tissue plane.

Example 14.3   ENT summary – letter form

> Thank you for referring this 69-year-old man to our ENT Clinic. He complains of poor hearing in his left ear for the last six months. Sounds appear muffled in that ear. The symptoms occurred during a heavy cold and have never resolved. He has no **otorrhoea** or pain in the ear and no history of dizziness or **tinnitus**. He is a diet-controlled diabetic and has had problems with varicose ulcers. He smokes 12 cigarettes a day.
>
> On examination his left tympanic membrane is struck down on to the *promontory* and there is a large retraction pocket in the drum. This means that there is very little air in the middle ear and the eardrum cannot vibrate in response to sound. Examination of the right ear shows mild retraction only.
>
> On examination of the nose there was a purulent discharge in the right nostril and on further questioning it appears that the patient has had sinus trouble for many years. Plain tone **audiogram** shows a 40 **decibel** hearing loss in the right ear which is of **sensory neural** origin and a 60 decibel loss in the left year which although mainly sensory neural, has an added **conductive** component. It therefore appears that he is suffering from Eustachian tube dysfunction on the left side, probably secondary to infected sinuses. He also has an element of **presbycusis**. I have prescribed some Otrivine nose drops to use in the left nostril in an attempt to open up his Eustachian tube. He is also having some sinus X-rays. I will review him in two weeks' time.

Explanation of terms used in Example 14.3

audiogram chart of the variations of hearing of an individual. Audiometry is the testing of the sense of hearing; it may be plain tone or pure tone audiometry. Acoustic impedance measurement is another test carried out, especially on those suspected of having fluid in the middle ear.

decibel   a unit used to express intensity of sound; abbreviation: dB.

otorrhoea   discharge from the ear.

presbycusis   a bilateral progressive perceptive deafness occurring with age, may be called senile deafness.

promontory   projecting process or eminence.

sensory neural   a form of deafness. Other forms include: conductive, perceptive, arteriosclerotic or otosclerotic deafness.

tinnitus   noises in the ear such as ringing, buzzing, roaring, clicking etc.

Example 14.4   ENT summary – letter form

> Thank you for referring this 75-year-old lady who has apparently had bilateral tinnitus since her ears were syringed in June. She feels that this is much better now but is still present to a slight extent. In addition she gets occasional rotatory **vertigo** and had bilateral epistaxis four days ago.
>
> On examination her tympanic membranes are healthy. She had a deviated nasal septum to the right and there were prominent vessels in both **Little's areas**. Pure tone audiometry reveals a hearing level of 50–60 decibels on the right side and 30–60 decibels on the left. **Tympanometry** was normal.
>
> Her Little's areas were cauterized with silver nitrate. She does not want a hearing aid. I have explained that there is nothing further we can do for her tinnitus but we will see again in four months' time because of her vertigo. At the present time I do not think further investigations are indicated.

Explanation of terms used in Example 14.4

Little's areas   anterior part of the nasal septum that is richly supplied with blood vessels and is often a common site for nose bleeds (sometimes called Kiesselbach's area).

tympanometry   a test to assess the function of the middle ear.

vertigo   a sensation of dizziness commonly due to disease or disturbance of the inner ear.

Example 14.5   ENT summary – letter form

> Thank you for referring this unfortunate boy who is asthmatic and sneezes daily. Over the past six months he has had a constantly blocked nose with nasal discharge and an aggravation of his asthma.
>
> He sleeps very poorly and wakes gasping for breath, not being able to breathe through his nose. He is also a noisy mouth breather.
>
> X-rays of his sinuses today revealed a marked **mucosal thickening** in both maxillary antra, worse on the left side with small **adenoids**.   →

Clinical examination of his nose revealed evidence of sinusitis with **mucopus** in both nasal chambers. He has very unhealthy looking tonsils with palpable **tonsillar cervical lymph nodes** and there is a past history of a lot of tonsillitis. Luckily his middle ears were clear and there is no history of **otitis media**.

This child probably has a bilateral maxillary sinusitis, possibly combined with nasal allergy, in view of his asthma. He should benefit from having his unhealthy tonsils and adenoids removed coupled with a sub-mucous diathermy (SMD) to both inferior turbinates to improve the nasal airways and a bilateral maxillary sinus washout with passage of in-dwelling tubes to both maxillary antra, if required, to facilitate daily sinus washouts.

It will be interesting to see how much better he is in terms of his nose, sinuses and chest in the postoperative period. Should there be any residual nasal allergy, we can cope with it after he is infection-free.

In the meantime I have requested our speech therapist to send for him with a view to any advice and treatment she can offer for his hoarse voice which is due to moderate size vocal nodules. He is an excitable child prone to screaming and shouting and at some later stage I will place him for **microlaryngoscopy** and stripping of both **vocal cords** should his hoarseness not improve significantly with speech therapy.

Explanation of terms used in Example 14.5

adenoids thickening (hypertrophy) of the adenoid tissue which normally exists in the nasopharynx of children.

microlaryngoscopy looking down the throat with the aid of a laryngoscope.

otitis media infection of the middle ear.

mucosal thickening thickening of mucous membrane (mucosa).

mucopus mucus looking like pus.

tonsillar cervical lymph nodes swollen glands in the neck due to infected tonsils.

vocal cords fold of mucous membrane in the larynx.

Example 14.6   ENT summary – letter form

This man recently underwent a **SMR** operation with trimming of his **inferior turbinates**. After an initial intranasal **synechia** which has now been divided, he has derived great benefit from the procedure.

He is now attending because of his ear problems. He has had a right tympanic perforation (posterior inferior marginal) ever since childhood and he is aware of right-sided deafness, an inability to locate sound or to hear in the presence of background noise.

Luckily he has never had any right-sided otorrhoea. At the moment in the right ear there is mixed deafness with hearing levels averaging the 55 decibel mark.

→

> The remainder of his tympanic membrane is chalky and tympanosclerotic but his **ossicular chain** appears to be intact. I have consequently placed him on my waiting list to have a right-sided tympanoplasty type I operation carried out.

Explanation of terms used in Example 14.6

inferior turbinates one of three turbinate bones (superior, middle and inferior) at the back of the nose. Trimming of the inferior turbinates is done to improve the nasal airway.

ossicular chain the three ossicles (small bones in the middle ear, the malleus, incus and stapes).

SMR operation submucous resection: nose operation done in cases of chronic nasal congestion and rhinitis.

synechia adhesion of parts, sometimes occurs after the inferior turbinates operation.

Glossary of other ENT terms

Term	Meaning
anosmia	absence of the sense of smell.
attic	cavity on wall of the tympanic membrane.
barotrauma	injury due to excessive pressures usually to structures of the ear.
Bell's palsy	facial paralysis due to lesion of the facial nerve.
cerumen	ear wax.
choana	the paired openings between the nasal cavity and nasopharynx.
cholesteatoma	cyst-like mass commonly occurring in the middle ear and the mastoid region.
concha	hollow of the auricle of the external ear.
coryza	common cold.
diplacusis	perception of a single auditory stimulus as two separate sounds.
gasserian	trigeminal (5th cranial nerve) ganglion.
helicotrema	passage at the apex of the cochlea.
labyrinthitis	otitis interna causing vertigo and vomiting.
Menière's disease	disease of the inner ear causing vertigo and progressive deafness.
ozena	atrophic rhinitis.
Rinne's test	hearing test with tuning fork: positive in normal hearing or sensory neural deafness, negative in conductive deafness.
sialadenitis	inflammation of a salivary gland.

Term	Meaning
tragus	cartilaginous projection anterior to the external opening of the ear.
utricle	the larger of the two divisions of the membranous labyrinth.
Valsalva's manoeuvre	forcible exhalation against closed nostrils and mouth causing increased pressure in Eustachian tubes and middle ear.
Weber's test	hearing test with tuning fork, result may be referred to as central, right or left.

Ear nose and throat operations

Name	Procedure

Ear procedures

fenestration	surgical creation of a new opening in the labyrinth for restoration of hearing in cases of otosclerosis.
mastoidectomy	excision of the mastoid cells or mastoid process.
myringotomy	surgical incision of the tympanic membrane.
ossiculoplasty	repair of the ossicles in the ear.
repair perforated tympanic membrane with Silastic splinting	self explanatory.
stapedectomy	excision of the stapes.
tympanoplasty	surgical reconstruction of the hearing mechanism in the middle ear.
tympanotomy	incision of the tympanic membrane.

Nose procedures

adenoidectomy	surgical removal of adenoids (pharyngeal tonsil) – increase in glandular tissue in the nasopharynx which normally exists in children.
correction of deviated nasal septum	the nasal septum is a plate of bone and cartilage covered with mucous membrane which divides the nasal cavity. Injury or malformation can produce a deviated septum causing nasal obstruction.
exploration of post-nasal space	exploration of the paranasal sinuses behind the nose usually because of infection.
nasal polypectomy	removal of polyps (mass with a stalk protruding from skin or mucous membrane) in the nasal cavity usually caused by local irritation or allergy, may cause nasal obstruction but are not malignant.

Name	*Procedure*
rhinoplasty	plastic surgery to the nose.
submucous diathermy (SMD)	diathermy to the mucous membrane of the nasal passages.
submucous resection (SMR)	surgical procedure to relieve obstruction, irritation and infection in the nose and sinuses.
trimming of inferior turbinates	modification of the turbinate bones – the upper, middle and lower conchae bones.

Sinus procedures

antral washout	a procedure to wash out the antrum or maxillary sinus. Some other related phrases that may occur are bilateral antral washouts (BAWO) and diagnostic bilateral maxillary sinus washouts.
Caldwell-Luc operation	a procedure to place an opening into the maxillary sinus in order to remove diseased membrane linings of the maxillary sinus.
intranasal antrostomy	a procedure to drain the sinus of a patient who suffers repeated attacks of acute maxillary sinusitis or who fails to respond to antibiotics and antral washouts.

Throat procedures

cricopharangeal myotomy	cutting the muscles of the cricoid cartilage and pharynx.
laryngectomy	surgical removal of the larynx.
laryngoscopy (micro-, direct, or indirect)	examination of the larynx.
tonsillectomy	surgical removal of a tonsil.
Ts and As	tonsils and adenoids
stripping of vocal cords	
tracheostomy	an opening in the neck giving access for the throat and insertion of an in-dwelling tracheostomy tube so patient can breathe.
tracheotomy	surgical incision in the windpipe (trachea) to allow the patient to breathe despite blockage.

Chapter 15
Gynaecology, Obstetrics, and Paediatrics

Gynaecology, obstetrics and paediatrics have been put together in one chapter because of the overlap of some terminology such as early complications of pregnancy and neonatal abnormalities. For basic anatomy, see Chapter 5.

Gynaecological and obstetric reports are followed by common abbreviations, useful terms and list of operations. Paediatric reports are followed by some paediatric abnormalities and conditions requiring operation.

Examples of gynaecology summaries with explanations of terms used

Example 15.1   Gynaecology summary – letter form

Thank you for referring this 49-year-old lady complaining of **menorrhagia**. Her periods are normally regular, cycle 5/28. However in March this year her period was heavier than normal followed by spotting for one month. Then in May her period was heavy and lasted 18 days and did not stop until she was started on Primolut N by you. She has had no intermenstrual bleeding, **post-coital bleeding** or **dyspareunia**. She had a normal cervical smear in June. She has no menopausal symptoms. Bowels and micturition NAD. She was seen about ten years ago by a gynaecologist and told that she had fibroids.

Past obstetric history: Para 2 + 1 [two normal vaginal deliveries and a miscarriage].

On examination she was well, abdomen soft, tip of uterus palpable. Vaginal examination – vulva and vagina normal, cervix – **polyp in os**, uterus **anteverted, 10–12 weeks' size**, mobile, **adnexa** NAD.

We have arranged for her to come in for a **D&C** and polypectomy. We are also checking her full blood count today. We are also stopping her **norethisterone** but obviously if she should get heavy bleeding she will need to restart it. I have warned her that she may need a hysterectomy eventually.

Explanation of terms used in Example 15.1

adnexa refers to uterine appendages, ovaries, tubes and ligaments.

anteverted normal position for the uterus.

D&C dilatation and curettage: common gynaecological procedure involving gentle dilatation of the cervix followed by scraping of the inside of the uterus.

dyspareunia painful intercourse.

menorrhagia excessive menstrual loss.

norethisterone a synthetic progesterone (a progestogen); a component of some oral contraceptive pills and compounds, as here, to control heavy menstrual bleeding.

para 2 + 1 two live births + one miscarrige.

polyp in os the cervix has an internal and external os. This is a common site for polyps.

post-coital bleeding bleeding after intercourse.

5/28 convention for expressing time – i.e. 5 days, every 28/month.

10–12 weeks' size uterus is measured by gestational size, i.e. the size the uterus would be if the patient was 10–12 weeks' pregnant.

Example 15.2   Gynaecology summary – letter form

I would be grateful for your help with this patient. She is aged 45 and has had four children. She originally had a total hysterectomy and Birch colposuspension when histology showed **adenomyosis**.

Her symptoms of frequency, **stress incontinence** and a dragging sensation were then relieved until last year. She now suffers from an unpleasant dragging/pressure sensation from the bladder, slight stress incontinence and frequency of micturition. There is no nocturia. Her main problem however is leaking of urine when she walks such that it is a considerable trouble and embarrassment.

Examination shows a **urethrocoele** and anterior prolapse either side of the original colposuspension which is clearly still supporting her vagina. **Urodynamic studies** have been reported as suggesting a low urethral pressure profile. I would greatly appreciate your opinion and expertise in advising her and carrying out further surgery if this would be the answer.

Explanation of terms used in Example 15.2

adenomyosis a benign condition characterized by ingrowth of the endometrium (lining of the uterus).

stress incontinence incontinence of urine caused by pressure such as coughing, sneezing, laughing, or exercise.

urethrocoele prolapse of the female urethra through the meatus.

urodynamic studies studies normally carried out in Clinical Measurement using a catheter into the bladder and saline infusions for assessing bladder tone and capacity.

Examples of obstetric summaries with explanations of terms used

Example 15.3   Ante-natal booking letter

Normally patients book at the hospital at about 14 weeks of pregnancy and if all is normal, care is shared with the patients' general practitioners.

> Thank you for referring this patient for booking. She is now ten weeks' pregnant. Although she was a little disappointed that we could not arrange any competent cardiac scan before 18 weeks, as the fetal heart is simply not large enough to check for abnormalities, we have arranged this investigation at the appropriate time. The only extra checks are the serum **AFP** at 16 weeks and a scan at 16 and 20 weeks for other fetal abnormalities.
>
> Her brother has **autism** but has not yet had a chromosome analysis. This she feels she would like to arrange so that if her brother is suffering from fragile X mental retardation, then she would like **amniocentesis** carried out. If all these investigations are normal then we would be happy to **share care** and indeed not to see her again until 28 weeks.

Explanation of terms used in Example 15.3

AFP   alphafetoprotein, a substance produced by the fetus. Raised levels associated with neural tube defects such as spina bifida.

amniocentesis   an investigation where a needle is inserted through the abdominal wall and amniotic fluid is withdrawn for chromosome analysis. Frequently performed in women over 38 years or where there is a history of Down's syndrome or other chromosome defect. Cannot be carried out before 16–18 weeks' gestation and not without risk of miscarriage.

autism   a condition of children characterized by failure to relate to people in the normal way and language disorders.

share care   referring to 'shared care' scheme whereby antenatal care shared by both GP and local consultant unit.

Example 15.4   Post-natal letter

Every newly-delivered mother has a post-natal check up at about six weeks.

> This patient came for a post-natal check up following a Caesarean section which was on account of **fetal distress** occurring on top of severe **pre-eclampsia**. The Caesarean section was six weeks ago and she has made a good recovery despite still getting some pain in the right side of her abdominal wound. As she has put on a considerable amount of weight I have referred her to the dietician. Contraception will be by Durex.
>
> Her blood pressure was 125/80 and urine testing was clear. I have advised her to ensure she doesn't fall pregnant for six months to allow the wound to
>
> →

heal up well. I have not arranged to see her again. Under ideal conditions with a spontaneous labour she could in future, be allowed a trial of scar and may achieve a vaginal delivery. However, with the severity of symptoms which she had before, we would tend to advise an elective Caesarean section. These matters must be left open to be decided upon at the appropriate time.

Explanation of terms used in Example 15.4

fetal distress is detected by listening to the baby's heart rate with a trumpet or by the cardiotocograph (CTG) machine. This monitors the fetal heart during contraction, giving a tracing. Increasingly used during most labours.

labour there are three stages:

1st from onset of regular contractions to the cervix being fully dilated at 10 cm.

2nd from full cervical dilation to the birth of the baby.

3rd from birth of the baby to delivery of the placenta and membranes followed by contraction of the uterus.

pre-eclampsia is a serious condition arising during pregnancy (especially first ones) characterized by raised blood pressure, protein in the urine (proteinuria), and oedema. No known cause, though dietary factors seem implicated. If unchecked can lead to eclampsia with seizures.

Abbreviations in gynaecology and obstetrics

Some of these have been included in the list at the end of Chapter 9 but for reference purposes it was thought helpful to list them again.

AFP	alpha-fetoprotein, a blood test to detect neural tube defects in fetus.
AID/AIH	artificial insemination donor/husband.
ANC	antenatal clinic.
APH	antepartum haemorrhage.
ARM	artificial rupture of membranes.
CVS	chorionic villus sampling.
D&C	dilatation and curettage.
DUB	dysfunctional uterine bleeding.
EDC	expected date of confinement.
EDD	expected date of delivery.
ERPC	evacuation of retained products of conception.
EUA	examination under anaesthetic.
FH	fetal heart.
FHR	fetal heart rate.
HVS	high vaginal swab.
IU(C)D	intrauterine (contraceptive) device.

IUD	intrauterine death (though also intrauterine device).
IVF	*in vitro* fertilization.
LMP	last menstrual period.
LOA/ROA	left or right occipitoanterior (positions of fetal head).
LSCS	lower segment Caesarean section.
NND	neo-natal death.
NVD	normal vaginal delivery.
OP	occipitoposterior (position of fetal head).
PID	pelvic inflammatory disease.
PMB	postmenopausal bleeding.
POC	products of conception.
POP	persistent occipitoposterior (abnormal position of fetal head in labour).
SB	stillborn.
STOP	suction termination of pregnancy.
TAH	total abdominal hysterectomy.
TOP	termination of pregnancy.

Glossary of gynaecology and obstetrics terms

Term	*Meaning*
abortion	loss of fetus. Some types are:

	habitual	= when there have been more than three miscarriages
	incomplete	= miscarriage with tissue left behind
	septic	= infection follows usually incomplete spontaneous or surgical abortion
	spontaneous	= miscarriage
	therapeutic	= induced termination of pregnancy.

abruptio placentae	premature separation of normally situated placenta.
amenorrhoea	absence of periods (may be primary where there have never been any, or secondary where they have stopped).
breech presentation	the baby is bottom-down and likely to be born bottom first.
chorionic villus sampling (CVS)	chorion is the outermost of the fetal membrane. A sample can be taken vaginally in early pregnancy (8–12 weeks) to detect chromosome abnormalities, rather than performing amniocentesis later (16–18 weeks).

Term	Meaning
cryocautery	cold cautery.
episiotomy	surgical incision of the perineum to aid delivery; may be performed by midwife.
gravida	a pregnant woman. Gravida I = pregnant for the first time (primigravida); multigravida = pregnant for the third or more times.
hydatidiform mole	abnormal pregnancy resulting from a pathological ovum; potentially malignant.
hydramnios	excess of anmiotic fluid.
leukoplakia vulvae	greyish-white patches on the vulval mucosa which cause irritation and may be pre-cancerous.
liquor	(in obstetrics) refers to amniotic fluid.
lochia	discharge from the vagina after delivery (some is normal).
meconium	first stools passed by the newborn. Indicates fetal distress when present in the liquor during labour.
mittelschmerz	pain midway in menstrual cycle associated with ovulation.
nulliparous	woman who has not produced a viable offspring.
parity	para I = had one child; refers to women who have borne viable offspring.
Pfannenstiel incision	neat transverse incision within the 'bikini' line commonly used now in Caesarean sections and gynaecological abdominal operations.
placenta praevia	placenta in the lower uterine segment, partially or entirely covering the internal os; serious condition.
pudendal block	local anaesthetic block of the pudendal nerve which numbs the vulval area.
puerperium	a period of about 6 weeks following childbirth when reproductive organs are returning to their normal state.
puerperal	pertaining to childbirth.
Shirodkar suture	Purse-string suture of cervix to prevent late miscarriage in those with a history of miscarrying. Performed at 14 weeks; removed at 36 weeks.
Stein-Leventhal syndrome	gynaecological condition associated with bilateral polycystic ovaries and infertility.

Term	Meaning
trachelorrhaphy	suture of the uterine cervix.
trimester	period of three months; there are three trimesters in pregnancy.

Obstetric forceps

Three obstetric forceps commonly used: Kielland; Neville Barnes; Wrigley.

Gynaecological operations

Name	Procedure
cerclage of cervix	putting a suture around the cervix (usually 'Shirodkar') in pregnancy in those who have a history of frequent late miscarriages.
colpoperineorrhaphy	repair of vagina and perineum.
colporrhaphy	repair of vagina: anterior for correction of cystocoele; posterior for correction of rectocoele.
colposcopy	examining the vagina and cervix by a colposcope and probably treating abnormal areas by laser.
colposuspension	operation for vaginal prolapse.
cone biopsy	removal of part of the cervix, done in some cases of abnormal cervical smears.
dilat(at)ion and curettage (D&C)	dilating the cervix to permit scraping of the walls of the uterus.
hysterectomy	removal of the uterus, may be: total abdominal (TAH) subtotal vaginal Wertheim's (radical excision performed to eradicate cervical cancer).
hysterosalpingogram	X-ray examination of the uterus and Fallopian tubes where contrast fluid is injected to ascertain if the tubes are patent in infertility investigations.
laparoscopic clip tubal occlusion	type of sterilization.
laparoscopy	examination of the pelvic cavity via a laparoscope which is inserted through a very small incision just under the umbilicus.
marsupialization of Bartholin's cyst	forming a pouch to treat an enclosed cyst in this area.
myomectomy	removal of fibroids from the uterus.
ovarian cystectomy	removal of ovarian cyst.

Name	*Procedure*
salpingoophorectomy	removal of Fallopian tubes and ovaries.
termination of pregnancy (TOP)	surgical abortion.
tubal ligation	type of sterilization.

Examples of paediatric summaries with explanations of terms used

Example 15.5   Paediatric summary – letter form

I saw this baby today at 15 weeks' old (9 weeks when corrected for prematurity). His case is complicated and there have been many problems.

1 **Preterm** *low birth weight (***GA** *34 weeks,* **BW** *1.72 kg)*
First pregnancy. Uneventful to 34 weeks. Emergency Caesarean section on account of **pv** bleeding and early labour. Birth weight below the 10th centile.

2.   *Birth asphyxia*
Apgars 2 at 1, 2 at 5 and 6 at 10 minutes. **Intubated** at six minutes, Extubated at ten minutes. Continuing respiratory difficulties. Re-intubated and ventilated from 20 minutes. First blood gases at 60 minutes showed acidosis and base deficit, pH 7.03, base deficit 17.

3.   *Surfactant deficiency and* **bronchopulmonary dysplasia**
Artificial ventilation from 20 minutes of age. Chest X-ray typical of **surfactant** deficiency with 'white out'. Ventilation for 8 days maximum pressure 24/4, maximum oxygen requirement 60%. Continuing oxygen dependency and respiratory distress after extubations. In air day 33.

4.   *Cleft lip and palate – partial trisomy chromosome 13*
Cleft lip and palate noted at birth. Subsequent chromosome analysis shows **partial trisomy** of the long arm 13. He was seen by the consultant geneticist who could find no other dysmorphic features and felt that the cleft was in keeping with the chromosome results. Literature search showed no exactly similar case and it is not possible to predict long term neurodevelopmental outcome. Nevertheless this will be followed closely.

5.   *Neonatal seizures*
The baby had three generalized seizures on the second and third days of life. These were treated with phenobarbitone and subsequently ceased. Initial cranial ultrasound (day 1) was normal but repeat on day 14 showed possible periventricular **leukomalacia** on the right. Other investigations were negative and the fits were ascribed to **birth asphyxia**.

6.   **Hyperbilirubinaemia**
Maximum bilirubin 225. **Phototherapy**. Investigations negative.

7.   *Abdominal distension – suspected* **NEC**
Abdominal distension with bile-stained aspirates occurred on day 5 but abdominal X-rays were normal. He was treated with **PPN** to day 16 and →

received triple antibiotic therapy for seven days. Feeds were subsequently introduced without problem.

8. *Bradycardias*
Series of **bradycardias** associated with cyanosis on day 28. Investigations negative. Treated with theophylline. Settled.

9. *Closure of lip at 9 weeks*
Surgery undertaken uneventfully but postoperative collapse required emergency resuscitation. Damage to surgical closure but no further surgery is necessary at the present time.

10. *Further cyanotic episodes at week 13*
Re-admitted at 13 weeks following a series of **cyanotic spells** at home. Further attacks in hospital appeared to be seizures.
Investigations (csf, plasma and urine aminoacids, urine metabolic screen, repeat ultrasound and EEG) all unhelpful. Discharged on phenobarbitone with apnoea monitor.

When I saw him today the picture was, in fact, encouraging. His length, weight and head circumference have all increased sharply recently and lie within the normal standards for his corrected age. His feeding is much improved and he now feeds from an ordinary bottle and teat. Feeds are quickly taken. He has recently started smiling and laughing and he fixates and follows. Mother is less sure that he hears normally.

On examination he looked well and there were no additional findings. The repair of his lip is reasonable. He has an umbilical hernia which will close spontaneously. Examination of heart and lungs was normal.

I plan to review his case in two months' time. He should remain on phenobarbitone 10 mg bd, but if his progress is satisfactory I intend to stop anticonvulsants at this point.

I have arranged an audiology assessment. He should remain on iron and vitamin supplements until he is weaned. Because of his history of neonatal seizures and cyanotic attacks which may have been fits, **pertussis** immunization is contraindicated, although immunization later in childhood can be reconsidered at a later date.

His parents have been given full details of his illness and have been told about the chromosome defect. The long-term outlook is uncertain but after todays's consultation I am encouraged about his progress.

Explanation of terms used in Example 15.5

Apgar score is a score which measures the baby's heart rate, muscle tone, respirations, reflex and colour immediately after delivery. A good score is 8 at 1 min, 9 at 5 min and 10 at 10 min. This baby has a very low score denoting birth asphyxia, which can be due to many causes – a difficult birth and prematurity being two.

apnoea cessation of breathing. An apnoea monitor is often supplied to parents with a previous history of 'cot death', now more commonly called sudden infant death syndrome (SIDS).

birth asphyxia   the baby does not start to breath spontaneously and has to be resuscitated.

BW (birth weight)   baby's weight at birth is an indicator of health.

bradycardia   slow heart rate.

bronchopulmonary dysplasia   is a condition in the lungs often found (together with surfactant deficiency) in premature babies sometimes referred to as respiratory distress syndrome (RDS) or hyaline membrane disease. This baby was nursed in an incubator and was able to be put in a normal cot 'in air' on day 33.

cyanotic attack   suddenly becoming blue, due to lack of oxygen.

dysmorphic feature   feature not in keeping with the totally normal make-up.

GA (gestational age)   term is 40 weeks' gestation. Birth at 34 weeks' gestational age means that the baby is pre-term – i.e. premature. The corrected age is the age the baby would have been if born at term.

hyperbilirubinaemia   excess of bilirubin, a bile pigment. Common condition in many newborn babies causing jaundice. Treatment is by phototherapy.

intubated   a tube is inserted into the trachea for ventilation. Extubated is removal of the tube. Most babies at birth require pharyngeal suction and some need oxygen by face mask but normally this is sufficient. The baby is intubated when there are severe breathing difficulties.

leuko-   white substance of the brain.

malacia   softening.

NEC   necrotizing enterocolitis – a serious intestinal condition affecting mainly premature babies.

neonatal   new born period. Newly born babies sometimes referred to as neonates.

partial trisomy chromosome 13   trisomy is the presence of an additional chromosome often causing abnormality.

pertussis   whooping cough.

phototherapy   babies are put under an ultraviolet lamp for a certain period daily until the jaundice resolves.

PPN   peripheral parenteral nutrition – intravenous feeding.

pv bleeding   vaginal bleeding. A Caesarean section is normally performed as a precaution in cases of early labour with pv bleeding.

seizures   fits.

surfactant   special substance in the lungs necessary allowing for elasticity and the exchange of gases.

Example 15.6   Paediatric summary – letter form

Thank you very much for referring this boy, diagnosed as **mosaic** 46XY/ 46XO genotype, probably mixed **gonadal dysgenesis**. I note from the past history that he had removal of uterus, tubes and a gonad during a right herniotomy in infancy, when he was also noted to have a partial bifid   →

scrotum; he has had serial repairs for penile scrotal **hypospadias** and he has had orchidopexy for his previously undescended left gonad, which appears to have had the histology of a testis, when biopsied in infancy.

At 10 4/12 years of age his height of 124.6 cm is below the 3rd centile but seems to represent reasonable growth velocity over the past few months; he clearly however, warrants full endocrine investigations and I have arranged for him to come in as a day case for assessment of his **hypothalamic**, pituitary, gonadal and adrenal axis as well as **HCG** testing, ultrasound scans and repeat of chromosomes. I shall see him in a few weeks with the results.

Explanation of terms used in Example 15.6

genotype   genetic constitution; *karotype* = chromosomal constitution.

gonadal dysgenesis   defective development of gonads (here, testes)

HCG   human chorionic gonadotrophin, a hormone.

hypospadias   congenital penile defect in which urinary opening is on the underside of penis. Corrected surgically.

hypothalamic   referring to the hypothalamus of the brain which regulates secondary sex characteristics and hormones (as well as water balance, food intake, temperature and sleep).

mosaic   genetic term meaning that an individual has two or more cell lines which are distinct (mosaic pattern).

Paediatric operations

Operations may be required in the newborn for congenital defects. Some will need to be done urgently while others can wait until the baby is older.

Children of course may need other operations, common to adults, and these are mentioned in the relevant chapters – including plastic surgery procedures to correct some congenital abnormalities.

Congenital abnormalities requiring surgery

Heart defects

There are many variations:

Fallot's tetralogy   is a combination of four heart defects

TGV   stands for transposition of the great vessels.

Patent ductus arteriosus (PDA)   is an open lumen in the ductus arteriosus, between the aorta and pulmonary artery after birth. It often closes with medication but if it persists it is usually corrected by surgery later.

Hydrocephaly

Accumulation of fluid in the cranial vault causing a large head. Insertion of a valve and shunt (Spitz Holter valve) may be used to relieve this condition.

Hydronephrosis

Distension of the calyces and pelvis of the kidney with urine. This is usually because of absence or obstruction of the ureter. Treated surgically.

Hypospadias

Hypospadias is a development anomaly in the male where the urethra does not open at the tip of the penis. It may be coronal, glandular or penile.

Epispadias can occur in either sex and is absence of the upper wall of the urethra. Chordee is the downward deflection of the penis seen in hypospadias.

Imperforate anus

The baby fails to pass meconium due to the anus being closed over and therefore this requires immediate surgery.

Oesophageal atresia

Atresia is the absence or closure of a normal body orifice or tubular organ. In the case of the oesophagus it is usually very serious and usually requires immediate surgery.

Omphalocoele

Protrusion of part of the intestines through a defect in the abdominal wall.

Pyloric stenosis

Narrowing of the pyloric orifice of the stomach. This causes projectile vomiting and is remedied by a simple operation called Ramstedt's operation.

Spina bifida

Defective closure of the spinal cord often with meningocoele (cystic protrusion of meninges) or myelomeningocoele (spinal cord and meninges).

Genitourinary operations

Meatotomy   incision of urinary meatus in order to enlarge it.

orchidopexy   bringing down and fixing of an undescended testis, usually done in two stages.

separation of congenital preputial adhesions   if these adhesions have not separated in young boys they may suffer recurrent attacks of balanitis which is infection of the prepuce (foreskin).

hydrocoele   collection of fluid in the tunica vaginalis which may occur in boys who have an inguinal hernia. Herniotomy is normally performed.

Abdominal operations

These may be performed for:

intussusception   infolding of one part of the intestine within another which leads to obstruction volvulus   twisting of the intestine

Hirschsprung's disease   an intestinal condition which may require investigations and biopsies to be undertaken under anaesthetic for diagnosis.

Chapter 16
Histopathology and Microbiology

Histopathology (with cytology) and microbiology are two of the specialist areas embraced by the field of pathology. Pathology is the study of disease (in all its aspects) and is laboratory-based (see Chapter 1). Histopathology deals with disease processes in tissues and organs and microbiology is the science of microorganisms, such as bacteria and viruses, many of which cause infection.

The secretary working in histopathology will find the dermatological glossary in Chapter 13 useful as well as the terms relating to tumours in Chapter 11.

The histopathology part of this chapter contains samples of histology reports, i.e. reports on the structure and composition of tissue sent for close examination. Some abbreviations used in the department and a list of useful terms are also included.

In the microbiology part, an alphabetical list of the commoner organisms causing disease in man is given. Note the italicization of some micro-organisms – this is the usual convention for genus and species names.

Examples of histopathology reports with explanations of terms used

The specimens are first examined by naked eye (described in the reports under the heading 'Macroscopy'); they are then classified for examination and in some cases the symbol α (alpha) is used. Following this they are examined under the microscope (Microscopy) by the histopathologist and a diagnosis given.

Example 16.1   Histology report

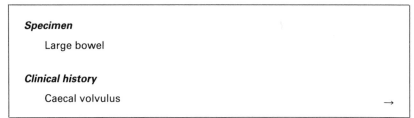

Specimen

Large bowel

Clinical history

Caecal volvulus   →

Macroscopy

Grossly dilated portion of thin-walled caecum, with 4 cm of descending colon and 9 cm irregular portion of terminal ileum. A 6 cm appendix is also included. The caecum was filled with soft faeces. The mucosa is moderately congested and contains **stercoral** ulcers around the ileocaecal valve region. No polyp or tumour seen.

Hist

    (A) Proximal resection margin × 1
    (B) Distal resection margin × 4 (3)
    (C) Rest × 6 (4)

Microscopy

Centrally the intestinal wall is oedematous and congested with haemorrhage and mucosal necrosis. The resection margins appear normal. The appendix has a fibrosed lumen.

Diagnosis

    Colon: consistent with volvulus, with viable ileal and colonic resection margins.

Explanation of terms used in Example 16.1

    stercolith (or faecolith)   an intestinal concretion formed round a centre of faecal material.
    stercoral faecal.

Example 16.2   Histology report

Specimen

    Products of conception (POC)

Clinical history

    Incomplete **abortion.**

Mascroscopy

Plentiful tissue fragments.

HIST α **all (2)**

      →

Microscopy

Inflamed haemorrhagic **decidua** with a few **chorionic villi** and **arias stella** secretory endometrium.

Diagnosis

Products of conception.

Explanation of terms used in Example 16.2

abortion   miscarriage. An incomplete miscarriage, with some products of conception left in the uterus is dangerous; there is a risk of both haemorrhage and infection.

arias stella reaction   a form of hypertrophy of the endometrium associated with the presence of chorionic tissue.

chorionic villi   thread-like projections over the external surface of the chorion, the outermost of the fetal membranes.

decidua   endometrium (lining of the uterus) during pregnancy.

Example 16.3   Histology report

Specimen

TUR (transurethral resection) of bladder tumour

Clinical history

Bladder tumour

Macroscopy

Multiple frond-like fragments of tissue up to 4 ml in volume

HIST α (2)

Microscopy

Papillary moderately differentiated transitional cell carcinoma infiltrating submucosa.
Some **pleomorphism** and only a few **mitoses** are seen.

Bladder biopsy

Infiltrative papillary moderately differentiated transitional cell carcinoma.

Explanation of terms used in Example 16.3

mitosis   the ordinary process of cell division which results in the formation of two daughter cells, and by which the body replaces dead cells. The presence of lots of mitotic figures shows a rapidly growing tumour.

pleomorphism   the existence of different sizes and shapes of a single cell type that is a bad sign when related to a tumour.

Example of post-mortem report

Example 16.4   Post-mortem report

Cause of death and other autopsy findings:

1. Acute myocardial infarction
2. Thrombosis of coronary artery
3. Atherosclerosis

External appearance

The body was that of a well nourished elderly Caucasian male weighing 80 kg.

Cardiovascular system

The pericardial sac was intact. The heart was heavy (540 g) due to left ventricular hypertrophy. The valves were unremarkable. There was an area of muscle scarring in the posterior wall of the left ventricle. The adjacent muscle was swollen and haemorrhagic. The coronary arteries were narrowed by atheroma. The right coronary artery contained an old occlusion and there was a fresh thrombus occluding the circumflex artery. The appearance was consistent with acute myocardial infarction.

Respiratory system

Unremarkable nasopharynx, larynx and trachea. The left pleural cavity was obliterated by fibrous adhesions. The lungs were heavy due to oedema. (right lung 800 g; left lung 750 g.)

Gastrointestinal system

Unremarkable mouth and oesophagus. There was a 4 cm mucus-filled diverticulum protruding into the peritoneal cavity at the gastro-oesophageal junction. The stomach, small and large intestine were unremarkable. The liver (1430 g) showed no underlying pathology. Unremarkable gall bladder, biliary duct system and pancreas.

Endocrine system

Unremarkable pituitary, thyroid and adrenal glands.   →

> ### Reticuloendothelial system
>
> Unremarkable lymph nodes and spleen (100 g).
>
> ### Urogenital system
>
> The kidneys showed no underlying pathology (right kidney 130 g, left kidney 120 g). Unremarkable ureters. The bladder was trabeculated consistent with bladder neck obstruction due to an enlarged nodular benign prostate gland. The testes were unremarkable. There was a hydrocoele on the right side.
>
> ### Central nervous system
>
> The brain showed no external or cut surface abnormality (1330 g). The cerebral vessels were patent. Normal meninges.

Histopathology terminology

Words to describe different types of cells and tissue are used widely in this speciality and most of these can be found in a comprehensive medical dictionary under *cell* or *tissue* but some are included here.

Term	Meaning
acinus	any of the smallest lobules of a compound gland (pl. acini).
amyloid	starch-like, an abnormal fibrillary protein deposited extracellularly in a variety of condtions.
argentaffin cell	type of cell found in the gastrointestinal tract.
atretic follicles	involuted ovarian follicles.
atypia	deviation from the normal or typical state.
Brunner's glands	glands in the submucosa of the duodenum.
Buerger's disease	disease affecting medium-size blood vessels, particularly in the arteries of the legs.
cancellous	spongy type of bone.
condylomata acuminata	viral wart-like lesions on the external genitalia or perianal region.
connective tissue	tissue that binds together, supports and protects. It consists of: fibrous tissue areolar tissue fat tendon cartilage bone.
cribriform	perforated like a sieve.

Term	Meaning
crypt	a blind pit or tube on a free surface.
dartoid	resembling the dartos (muscle under skin of scrotum).
ectasia	expansion, dilation or distension.
ectocervix	portion of the uterus that projects into the vagina.
enchondroma	benign tumour of cartilage.
endothelium	layer of epithelial cells lining the cavity of the heart, blood and lymph vessels.
epithelium	tissue that covers the external and internal surfaces of the body including the lining of vessels and other small cavities. Some types: ciliated columnar cuboidal squamous stratified transitional.
exophytic	growing outward, or tumour proliferating externally.
fascia	sheet or band of fibrous tissue, may be deep or subcutaneous.
fascicles	small bundles or clusters, especially of nerve or muscle fibres.
flocculent	containing downy or flaky shreds.
goblet cells	mucus-secreting cells found largely in the epithelium lining the respiratory tract, and large and small intestines.
haemosiderin	an insoluble form of storage iron.
helminth	parasitic worm.
histiocytes	scavenger cells (macrophages).
Hürthle cell	type of cell sometimes found in the thyroid gland.
intima	innermost coat of a blood vessel (e.g. tunica intima) (adj. intimal).
involucrum	covering or sheath. Used to describe sheath of new bone in cases of osteomyelitis.
Kupffer's cells	phagocytic cells found in the liver and part of the reticuloendothelial system.
lamina propria	connective tissue layer of mucous membrane.
LE cells	cells characteristic of lupus erythematosus.

Term	Meaning
leiomyomata	benign tumours of smooth muscle, usually refers to uterine fibroids.
Leydig's cells	interstitial cells of the testis.
lymphoid	pertaining to lymph or tissue of the lymphatic system.
lytic	referring to lysis (dissolution).
macrophages	mononuclear phagocytic cells which are components of the reticuloendothelial system. Digest cell debris and bacteria.
mast cells	large cells with large granules in the cytoplasm.
matrix	intercellular substance of a tissue, such as bone matrix.
mesenchymal	embryonic connective tissue.
mesothelium	layer of flat cells lining the body cavity of the embryo and in the adult forms the squamous epithelium which covers serous membrane, e.g. in the pleura, peritoneum and pericardium.
metaplasia	change in the type of adult cell in a tissue to a mature form abnormal to the tissue.
mycetoma	chronic disease caused by one of a variety of fungi, affecting usually hands, legs and feet.
myxoid	having a large acellular stromal component in which mucins are present.
oxyurid	pinworm, seatworm or threadworm.
parenchymatous	tissue forming the functional element of an organ.
psammoma bodies	microscopic calcareous material occurring in benign and malignant epithelial tumours.
pultaceous	pulpy.
pyknosis	a thickening, especially degeneration of a cell in which the nucleus shrinks in size and the chromatin condenses to a solid structureless mass (adj. pyknotic).
Reed-Sternberg cells	cells found in Hodgkin's disease.
rete	a network, or meshwork, especially of blood vessels.
Sertoli cells	cells found in the tubules of the testes.
sessile	not pedunculated, attached by a broad base.
sidero	word element, iron e.g. haemosiderosis.
squame	scale or thin plate-like structure.
unilocular	having only one loculus or compartment.

Some abbreviations in histology

bx	biposy.
c/s	cross section.
CT	connective tissue.
cx	cervix.
dec	decalcified.
EM	ellipse of mucosa or electron microscopy.
E/S	ellipse of skin.
FF	fibro-fatty.
FFT	fibro-fatty tissue.
F/S	frozen section.
HPV	human papilloma virus.
LN	lymph node.
MM	malignant melanoma.
PCs	prostatic chippings.
S/C sub-cut	subcutaneous.
sebic	seborrhoeic.
φ	diameter.

Glossary of terms used in microbiology

Microbiology is the study of microorganisms. Microorganisms causing infection in man are bacteria, fungi, protozoa, rickettsiae and viruses.

These microorganisms and the conditions caused by them are listed alphabetically and not, as would be more correct, in specific groups, to be of more help for reference purposes.

Some microorganisms are italicized with a capital letter; this is a strict convention which should be observed.

Term	*Meaning*
actinomycosis	fungi, sometimes found in wounds.
AIDS	acquired immune deficiency syndrome caused by the human immunodeficiency virus (HIV).
amoebic dysentry (amoebiasis)	intestinal infection caused by amoebae.
anthrax	caused by *Bacillus anthracis*, a type of bacteria. Acquired through infected animals.
aspergillosis	inflammatory granulomatous lesions caused by a genus of fungi (*Aspergillus*). Can affect lungs, skin, ear, orbit, sinuses and occasionally bone and meninges.
Bordetella	a type of bacteria that causes whooping cough.

Term	Meaning
Borrelia	a type of bacteria of which one form causes relapsing fever, transmitted by body lice.
botulism	extremely severe form of food poisoning caused by *Clostridium botulinum*.
brucellosis	undulant fever, caused by one or the various species of *Brucella*, a genus of bacteria.
candidiasis	infection by a fungi of the genus *Candida* usually *Candida albicans*. Can affect skin, oral mucosa, respiratory tract and vagina.
chickenpox	viral infection caused by varicella zoster virus (VZV).
Chlamydia	type of bacteria. Two species: *Chlamydia trachomatis* is one of most common sexually transmitted diseases and affects the eyes, urinary tract and cervix. *Chlamydia psittaci* infects birds and causes pneumonia in man.
cholera	caused by *Vibrio cholerae*, a genus of Gram-negative bacteria.
Clostridium	type of bacteria, many different species causing botulism, tetanus and gas gangrene.
Corynebacterium	a group of bacteria causing diphtheria and listeria.
diphtheria	severe infectious disease caused by *Corynebacterium diphtheriae*.
Enterobius vermicularis	threadworm.
Escherichia	a type of bacteria of the family enterobacteria. Pathogenic strain *E. coli* (coliform infection) causes urinary tract infections and in children epidemic diarrhoea.
Gardnerella	bacteria, *G. vaginalis* causes infection in the female genital tract.
gas gangrene	species of *Clostridium* causes this infection in contaminated wounds.
Giardia	protozoa, may cause protracted intermittent diarrhoea (giardiasis).
Giardia lamblia	a species parasitic in the intestine of man.
glandular fever	infectious mononucleosis, caused by Epstein-Barr virus.
gonococcus	bacteria of species *Neisseria gonorrhoeae* causing gonorrhoea.
Haemophilus	a genus of bacteria. *H. influenzae* can cause conjunctivitis, influenza, and meningitis.

Term	Meaning
hepatitis A	a virus causing infective hepatitis A. Slow-onset illness. virus spread by direct contact or faecal contamination.
hepatitis B	virus transmitted by contaminated blood causing serum hepatitis.
herpes simplex	virus, type 1 can cause cold sores and blisters, type 2 causes genital herpes.
herpes zoster	'shingles', caused by the same virus as chickenpox.
infectious mononucieosis	glandular fever.
influenza	caused by a virus of which there are many strains, three main types A, B and C.
Lactobacillus	a type of bacteria which may be related to dental caries but is otherwise non-pathogenic.
Legionella pneumophila	species of Gram-negative bacteria causing Legionnaires' disease.
leptospirosis	a group of notifiable diseases due to serotypes of *Leptospira*, a genus of bacteria; best known as Weil's disease spread through animals' urine, commonly rats.
Listeria	a type of bacteria of the family *Corynebacterium*. May cause upper respiratory disease, septicaemia and encephalitis and can harm the unborn baby.
malaria	caused by a protozoan parasite carried by mosquitoes.
measles	caused by a virus, also called morbilli or in English sometimes rubeola.
meningococcus	bacteria of the family *Neisseria*, causes some types of meningitis.
moniliasis	candidiasis or 'thrush'.
morbilli	measles.
mumps	caused by virus, may be called epidemic parotitis or parotiditis.
Mycobacterium	a type of bacteria, one form causes tuberculosis and another leprosy.
Mycoplasma	a type of bacteria, one species can cause pneumonia and another urethritis.
Neisseria	a type of bacteria, one form causing gonorrhoea and another meningitis.
pertussis	whooping cough, due to *Bordetella pertussis*.
phthisis	wasting of the body due to tuberculosis.

Term	Meaning
poliomyelitis	caused by the poliovirus.
Proteus	a genus of Gram-negative, motile bacteria usually found in faecal or putrefying matter, associated with summer diarrhoea and cystitis.
Pseudomas aeruginosa	a genus of Gram-negative bacteria which causes various human diseases.
psittacosis	an infection caught from parrots caused by *Chlamydia psittaci*.
rabies	caused by a virus belonging to the rhabdovirus group, often present in saliva of infected animals, e.g. dog, fox, and bat.
rhinovirus	a subgroup of the picorna viruses associated with the common cold and upper respiratory ailments.
rubella	German measles, caused by a virus which if contracted in early pregnancy can cause serious fetal abnormalities.
salmonella	any organism of the genus *Salmonella*, a bacteria which may be present in raw meat, poultry, eggs and dairy produce. Can cause abdominal cramps, diarrhoea and vomiting.
Shigella	a type of bacteria which causes dysentry
smallpox	also called variola. Serious infectious disease caused by the poxvirus which has been eradicated in the world since 1977.
Staphylococcus	a type of Gram-positive bacteria, most common cause of boils and wound infections. Some forms are S. *albus* (S. *epidermidis*) and S. *aureus*.
Streptococcus	type of Gram-positive cocci include the following groups: S. *pyogenes* (includes β-haemolytic streptococcus); S. *viridans* (includes α-haemolytic streptococcus); S. *faecalis*. Many diseases are caused by streptococci, including scarlet fever, rheumatic fever, erysipelas, and endocarditis.
syphilis	a venereal disease caused by a spiral shaped bacterium (spirochete) *Treponema pallidum*.
tetanus	caused by tetanus bacillus (*Clostridium tetani*), found in soil and dust especially in rural areas, spread by animal and human faeces. Also called 'lockjaw' because stiffness of the jaw is one of first symptoms.

Term	Meaning
tinea	ringworm, a fungal infection of the skin.
toxoplasmosis	a disease due to *Toxoplasma gondii*, a protozoan parasite in infected meat and cat faeces. The congenital form is extremely serious.
Trichomonas	a genus of flagellate protozoa parasitic in animals, birds and man, trichomoniasis is a sexually transmitted disease caused by *Trichomonas vaginalis*.
tuberculosis	an infectious disease commonly affecting the lungs, caused by the bacillus (*Mycobacterium tuberculosis*).
typhoid fever	a notifiable disease caused by bacteria, *Salmonella typhi*, transmitted by infected water, milk and other foods especially shellfish.
typhus	an acute notifiable infectious disease caused by species of the parasitic microorganism *Rickettsia* and usually lice borne.
varicella	chickenpox.
variola	smallpox.
whooping cough	pertussis.
Yellow fever	an acute notifiable infectious viral disease carried by mosquitoes, mainly in tropical America and Africa.
Yersina	a type of Gram-negative bacteria of the family Enterobacteriaceae. Transmitted to man from the rat flea, *Y. pestis* causes plague and *Y. pseudotuberculosis*, mesenteric lymphadenitis in man.

Chapter 17
Ophthalmology

A brief outline of the anatomy of the eye is given in Chapter 5. This chapter contains examples of ophthalmic summaries in letter form together with a list of eye operations and a comprehensive glossary of ophthalmological disease conditions and terms.

Examples of ophthalmology summaries with explanations of terms used

Example 17.1   Ophthalmic summary – letter form

Thank you for referring this patient who you will remember the optician suspected might have *glaucoma*.

On examination here today, testing showed the presence of a superior arcuate *scotoma* in the right field. The tensions were within normal limits and were not appreciably raised when her pupils were dilated. The discs may well be normal. On *gonioscopy*, the angles appear to be narrow with some pigment.

I would not like to make a diagnosis of glaucoma in this case but I think in view of the field findings we should keep her under close observation and I have asked her to come again is six months and to report immediately if she has any symptoms which could be attributable to closed angle glaucoma.

Explanation of terms used in Example 17.1

glaucoma   increase in pressure within the eye.
gonioscopy   measurement of the angle of the anterior chamber of the eye.
scotoma   an area of depressed vision surrounded by an area of normal or less depressed vision.

Example 17.2   Ophthalmic summary – letter form

> Thank you for referring this patient. Her *intraocular pressures* are 15 and 14 with some *nuclear sclerosis* and I felt the discs were within normal limits. As her intraocular pressures are so good, I am trying her with no drops for three months, just to see if there is any possibility of leaving her off them altogether. Our **Humphrey Field test** revealed no specific abnormality.

Explanation of terms used in Example 17.2

Humphrey Field test   a test to check visual fields, namely the extent of straightahead vision.

intraocular pressures   pressure within the eye.

nuclear sclerosis   hardening of the eye's lens; cataract.

Example 17.3   Ophthalmic summary – letter form

> I reviewed this patient who has been on antiglaucoma drops for several years. In fact her discs are normal and off treatment her intraocular pressures are satisfactory. I enclose a copy of her latest **Friedman fields**.
>
> She does have lens changes affecting both eyes, but her visual acuity is reasonable. I have asked her to be reviewed annually at the opticians, but she no longer needs to attend our clinic.

Explanation of terms used in Example 17.3

Friedman fields   test to check visual fields.

Example 17.4   Ophthalmic summary – letter form

> Thank you very much for sending the patient who I saw at the clinic today. She complains of blurring in the right eye for the past few years, worse in the last six months or so. Ocular examination revealed a visual acuity of counting fingers in the right eye and 6/12 in the left eye.
>
> The visual deficit in the right eye has been found to be due to *macular degenerative changes* in this eye. She has slight pigmentary changes in the left eye also, and she really needs a new pair of reading glasses which I have prescribed. With these the vision has been brought up to normal in the left eye. I could not unfortunately improve the right eye at all with any sort of glasses.
>
> I have reassured her and has asked her to come back in three months for a further check-up and prescribed Multivite tablets, one to be taken twice a day.

Explanation of terms used in Example 17.4

macular degenerative changes degenerative changes in the part of the retina responsible for accurate central vision.

Example 17.5   Ophthalmic summary – letter form

> This patient has been attending this clinic for the last four years. Previously she had a right *cataract operation* with *implant*. She had an immature cataract and *vitreous degeneration* in both eyes. Today her intraocular pressure was normal. She has 6/12 vision in the right eye and 6/18 in the left eye with her glasses.
>
> We have been following her up nine monthly and the picture remains much the same. We will review her again in nine months.

Explanation of terms used in Example 17.5

cataract operation removal of opaque lens and replacement with lens implant (see Operations).

vitreous degeneration vitreous = vitreous body, the transparent gel filling the inner portion of the eyeball between the lens and retina.

Example 17.6   Ophthalmic summary – letter form

> Many thanks for referring this patient whom I saw in the Eye Clinic today. He complained of difficulty with distance vision. On examination the visual acuity was 6/60 in each eye. This could be improved to 6/18 with appropriate myopic correction. He can manage small print without help of any glasses. Examination of the anterior segments revealed bilateral nuclear sclerosis. The intraocular pressures were at borderline, 26 in the right eye and 24 in the left. Both the fundi were normal. In particular there was no pathological **cupping of the optic disc**.
>
> In conclusion he has bilateral nuclear sclerosis with *lenticular myopia*. His cataracts do not require any action at this stage. He will be kept under review in the Eye Clinic.

Explanation of terms used in Example 17.6

cupping of the optic disc depression of the intraocular part of the optic nerve which appears as a pink to white disc in the retina.

lenticular myopia shortsightedness caused when the refractive power of the lens is too strong.

Example 17.7   Ophthalmic summary – letter form

> This child who was born at 33 weeks underwent ventriculoatrial shunting for obstructive hydrocephalus. He has never been noted to have any visual function.
>
> On examination he had asymmetric orbits, roving eye movements with no light fixation and a non-reactive right pupil. The left pupil did respond sluggishly.
>
> An examination under anaesthesia was performed which disclosed right *microphthalmos* with a corneal diameter of 7 mm on the right and 10.5 mm on the left. The right eye had extensive *pupillary remnants* with a pupillary membrane, and sectoral posterior cortical cataract. The right *fovea* was hypoplastic, the disc appeared dysplastic and a poor view of the retina was obtained, although this appeared to indicate that a retinal fold was present in the superior retina. The left eye showed fine pupillary remnants and markedly dysplastic optic disc with no detectable macula. The left eye had prominent vitreous base, but no evidence of regressed retinopathy of prematurity.

Explanation of terms used in Example 17.7

fovea   part of the retina.
microphthalmos   abnormal smallness in all aspects of the eye.
pupillary remnants   pupillary = pertaining to the pupil.

Glossary of ophthalmology terms and conditions

Term	Meaning
ablepharon	congenital reduction or absence of eyelid (adj. ablepharous).
accommodation	adjustment of the eye for focusing on object at various distances.
achromatopsia	complete inability to distinguish colours.
Adie's syndrome	a syndrome consisting of a pathological pupil reaction (pupillontonia).
amaurosis	loss of sight without apparent lesion of the eye e.g. from disease of the optic nerve.
amblyopia	reduced vision not due to organic defect.
ametropia	condition of the eye in which parallel rays fail to come to a focus on the retina (adj. ametropic).
angioscotoma	a defect in the visual field caused by the shadow of the retinal blood vessels.
aniseikonia	inequality of the size of the retinal images of the two eyes.
anisometropia	a considerable degree of inequality in the refractive powers of the two eyes.
ankyloblepharon	adhesion of the eyelids to each other.

Term	Meaning
anopsia	non-use or suppression of vision in one eye.
aphakia	absence of lens.
Argyll–Robertson pupil	pupil that is small and responds to accommodative effect but not to light; usually due to advanced syphilis.
asthenopia	weakness or easy fatigue of the eye with headaches (eye-strain).
astigmatism	error of refraction where no single focus is formed.
blepharitis	inflammation of the eyelids.
blepharoadenitis	inflammation of the meibomian glands of the eyelids.
blepharophimosis	abnormal narrowness of the palpebral fissures.
buphthalmos	abnormal enlargement of the eyes due to congenital glaucoma
canthoplasty	plastic surgery of a canthus.
canthus	the angular junction of the eyelids at either corner of the eyes.
capsulotomy	incision of the capsule of the lens.
cataract	opacity of the lens.
chalazion	small eyelid mass due to chronic inflammation of the meibomian gland (chalazion = hailstone).
chemosis	oedema of the conjunctiva of the eye.
choroid	part of the lining of the eye.
coloboma	an apparent absence or defect of some ocular tissue.
conjunctivitis	inflammation of the membrane covering the eyeball and lining the eyelids (conjunctiva).
convergence	the coordinated movement of two eyes towards fixation of the same near point.
corectopia	abnormal location of the pupil of the eye.
cornea	'white' of the eye.
cyclitis	inflammation of the ciliary body.
cyclophoria	a form of heterophoria – i.e. failure of the visual axes to remain parallel with one eye covered.
cycloplegia	paralysis of the ciliary muscle.
dacry(o)-	(word element) tears or the lacrimal apparatus of the eye.
dacryagogic	inducing a flow of tears or serving as a channel for discharge of secretions of lacrimal glands.
dacryoadenitis	inflammation of the lacrimal gland.
dacryocystitis	inflammation of the lacrimal sac.

Term	*Meaning*
dacryocystorhinostenosis	narrowing of the duct leading from the lacrimal sac to the nasal cavity.
dendritic ulcer	eye ulcer which may be caused by herpes simplex virus.
diplopia	double vision.
ectropion	turning outwards (eversion) of the margin of the eyelid.
endophthalmitis	inflammation of the ocular cavities and their adjacent structures.
entropion	inversion of the margin of an eyelid.
enucleation	removal of the eyeball.
epiphora	overflow of tears.
esotropia	form of squint (strabismus).
evisceration	(in ophthalmics) removal of the contents of the eyeball.
exophoria	form of squint (heterophoria).
exophthalmos	abnormal protusion of the eyeball.
fluorescein	a fluorescent dye used in solution to reveal corneal damage or foreign bodies in the eye.
fovea	small depression especially referring to the retina.
Friedman fields	test to check visual fields.
glaucoma	increase in intraocular pressure.
gonioscopy	examination of the angle of the anterior chamber of the eye with gonioscope.
hemianopia	loss of vision in half the visual field.
heterophoria	failure of visual axes to remain parallel after the fusional stimuli has been eliminated.
heterotropia	manifest squint.
hordeolum	stye.
Humphrey Field test	a test to check visual fields, namely the extent of straight ahead vision.
hypermetropia	long-sightedness.
hyperphoria	heterophoria in which there is upward deviation of the visual axis.
hyphema	haemorrhage into the anterior chamber of the eye.
hypopyon	pus in the anterior chamber of the eye.
intraocular pressure	pressure within the eye reflecting balance of the fluid of the aqueous humour. Imbalance causes raised intraocular pressure.
iridauxesis	thickening of the iris.
iridectomy	excision of part of the iris.

Term	*Meaning*
iridocyclitis	inflammation of the iris and ciliary body.
iridokeratitis	inflammation of the iris and cornea.
iridorhexis	rupture of the iris or tearing away of the iris.
irodoschisis	splitting of the mesodermal stroma of the iris into two layers.
iridosclerotomy	incision of the sclera and of the edge of the iris in glaucoma.
iridosteresis	removal of all or part of the iris.
keratectasia	protrusion of a thin scarred cornea.
keratitis	inflammation of the cornea.
keratoconus	conical protrusion of the central part of the cornea resulting in an irregular astigmatism.
keratoglobus	a bilateral anomaly in which the cornea is enlarged and globular in shape.
lacuna	a defect or gap as in the field of vision (scotoma).
lagophthalmos	inability to shut the eyelids completely.
lenticular	(in ophthalmics) pertaining to the lens of the eye.
macropsia	condition in which objects appear too large.
macula	the part of the retina that is responsible for accurate central vision.
madarosis	loss of eyelashes or eyebrows.
metamorphopsia	defective vision with distortion of objects looked at.
microphakia	abnormal smallness of the crystalline lens.
microphthalmos	abnormal smallness in all dimensions of an eye.
micropsia	disorder of visual perception in which objects appear smaller than their actual size.
miosis	constriction of the pupil.
miotic	an agent that causes constriction of the pupil.
mydriasis	dilatation of the pupil.
mydriatic	drug that dilates the pupil.
myopia	near-/short-sightedness.
neuroretinitis	inflammation of the optic nerve and retina.
nuclear sclerosis	term referring to a cataract, a hardening of the nucleus of the lens.
nyctalopia	night blindness.
nystagmus	involuntary rapid rhythmic movement of the eyeball.
ophthalmia	severe inflammation of the eye.
ophthalmoplegia	paralysis of the eye muscles.

Term	Meaning
ophthalmorrhoexis	rupture of an eyeball.
ophthalmoscope	instrument for examining the interior of the eye.
ophthalmosynchysis	effusion into the eye.
optic	of or pertaining to the eye.
orbit	bony cavity in skull containing the eyeball.
orthophoria	normal equilibrium of the eye muscles.
orthoptics	assessment and treatment of strabismus and related disorders.
orthoptist	one who specializes in the assessment and management of strabismus (squint).
palpebral fissure	longitudinal opening between eyelids.
pannus	superficial vascularization of the cornea with infiltration of granular tissue.
panophthalmitis	inflammation of all the eye structures or tissues.
papilloedema	non-inflammatory swelling of the optic nerve resulting from increased intracranial pressure.
photopsia	a sensation of sparks or flashes in retinal irritation.
photoretinitis	retinitis due to exposure to intense light.
pinguecula	small benign, yellowish spot on the bulbar conjunctiva seen usually in the elderly.
presbyopsia	diminution of accommodation of the lens of the eye occurring normally with ageing.
proptosis	bulging of the eye.
pterygium	wing-like structure, usually refers to an abnormal triangular fold of membrane in the interpalpebral fissure.
ptilosis	falling out of the eyelashes.
ptosis	drooping of the upper eyelid.
pupilla	pupil.
refraction	the determination of the refractive errors of the eyes and their correction with glasses.
retinitis	inflammation of the retina.
retinoblastoma	malignant tumour arising from retinal cells. Occurs in infancy and may be hereditary.
retinopathy	any non-inflammatory disease of the retina.
retinoschisis	splitting of the retina (juvenile and adult form occurring in different layers).
retrolental fibroplasia	retinopathy of prematurity (ROP).
scleritis	inflammation of the sclera.
scotoma	an area of depressed vision with the visual field surrounded by an area of normal or less depressed vision.

Term	Meaning
strabismus	squint or heterotropia. Various forms of squint referred to as tropias, their direction being indicated by appropriate prefix.
symblepharon	adhesion of the eyelid to the eyeball, resulting in obliteration of the fornices.
synchysis	a softening or fluid condition of the vitreous body of the eye.
synechia	adhesion, as of the iris to the cornea or the lens.
tarsoplasty	plastic repair of the tarsus.
tarsorrhaphy	suture of a portion of or the entire upper and lower eyelids.
tarsus	(in ophthalmics) cartilaginous plate forming the framework of upper or lower eyelids.
trachoma	chronic infectious disease of the conjunctiva and cornea.
trichiasis	ingrowing eyelashes.
uvea	the iris, ciliary body and choroid together. adj. uveal.
uveitis	inflammation of the uvea.
vitreous	vitreous body or humour, transparent gel filling the inner part of the eyeball.
yoked muscles	muscles acting simultaneously and equally, such as those moving the eyes.
zonule	small zone.
zonulitis	inflammation of the ciliary zonule.
zonulolysis	dissolution of the ciliary zonule by use of enzymes to permit surgical removal of the lens.
zonulysin	a proteolytic enzyme that may be used in eye surgery.

Some ophthalmological operations

Name	Procedure
capsulotomy	opening the capsule of the lens, commonly performed by laser, after cataract operation.
cataract operation	this is the surgical removal of the lens, lens extraction or cataract extraction. Extracapsule extraction is total removal of the lens within its capsule, intracapsular extraction is removal of

Name	Procedure
	the lens nucleus and cortex leaving the posterior lens capsule. Extracapsular cataract extraction and intracapsular lens implant, an operation commonly performed may be shortened to E/cat EXTN + IOL.
corneal grafting	keratoplasty. May be:

optic transplantation of corneal material to replace scar tissue

refractive removal of a section of cornea from patient (keratomileusis) or donor (keratophakia), then reshaped and sutured back to correct optical error.

tectonic transplantation of corneal material to replace tissue that has been lost.

Name	Procedure
dacryoadenectomy	excision of a tear (lachrymal or lacrimal) gland.
dacryocystectomy	excision of the wall of the lachrymal sac.
dacryocystorhinostomy	surgical creation of an opening between the lachrymal sac and nasal cavity.
enucleation	removal of an eyeball.
iridectomy	removal of a portion of the iris.
iridosclerotomy	incision of the sclera and of the edge of the iris performed for glaucoma.
radical keratotomy	operation in which a series of incisions are made in the cornea to flatten it in order to correct myopia.
tarsorrhaphy/ blepharorrhaphy	surturing together of portion of or entire upper and lower eyelids.

Chapter 18
Oral Surgery and Dentistry

The chapter contains some basic dental anatomy with a list of joints and muscles relevant to oral surgery. Explanations of dental terminology is given with samples of oral surgery reports and orthodontic letters. Examples of oral surgery operations and X-ray report of a parotid sialogram are also included.

In cases of severe facial injuries the oral and plastic surgeons work together as a team, one dealing with the bony and dental injuries and the other with the soft tissue damage and loss.

Basic dental anatomy

The first set of teeth are known as the deciduous teeth but are also referred to as baby, milk, temporary or primary teeth. There are 20 of them, 10 on each jaw. Figure 18.1 shows the deciduous teeth giving their names and designations.

The permanent teeth are the second and final set of teeth. There are 32 of them, 16 on each jaw. Figure 18.2 shows the permanent teeth along with their names and designations. Each tooth has a crown and a root. The crown, above the gum, is covered by enamel and the surface of the root is composed of cementum. The major portion of the tooth is formed of dentine and is solid except for a pulp cavity contained within, where there are nerves, blood and lymph vessels.

The dental alveoli are the sockets in the mandible in which the roots of the teeth are attached. Fibrous connective tissue, called the periodontium, covers the root of each tooth and helps to keep it in place as well as cushion it against pressure from biting and chewing.

The gum is known as the gingiva (pl. gingivae).

The *muscles of the jaw and face* (relevant to oral surgery) are:
buccinator
depressor anguli oris
depressor labii inferior
greater zygomatic
lateral and medial pterygoid
masseter
orbicularis oris
platysma
temporalis

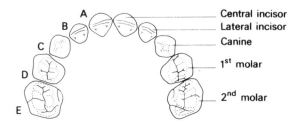

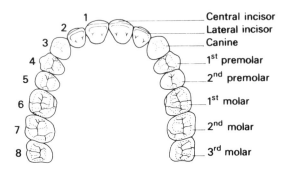

Fig. 18.1 The deciduous teeth. (*Source* Levison 1991.)

Fig. 18.2 The permanent teeth. (*Source* Levison 1991.)

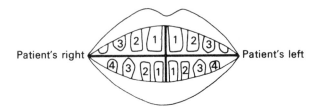

Fig. 18.3 Charting teeth. (*Source* Levison 1991.)

The *joints* are the:
  temporomandibular (often referred to as TMJs (temporo mandibular joints))
  temporomaxillary

Charting of teeth

When describing teeth they are numbered (permanent teeth) or lettered (deciduous teeth) from the centre backwards, see Fig. 18.3.

Teeth can be further divided into four groups or quadrants, according to their position in the mouth, and given a symbol to denote this position:

upper right   ⌐|

upper left |⌐

lower right   ⌐|

lower left |⌐

The secretary is reminded that in typing the position of teeth the right and left describes the patient's right and left not the dental surgeon's as he faces the patient.

So using this scheme the following symbols are translated:

|6   upper left first molar

3|3   upper left and upper right canines

$\frac{4|4}{4|4}$ all four first premolars

The secretary should also be aware of another system for identifying teeth. In view of the difficulties that may be experienced by the secretary in trying to get the department typewriter or word processor to type these symbols legibly the International Dental Federation has recommended that a two-digit system be adopted to allow easier presentation and transmission of data. The system replaces the four quadrants with a number:

Old quadrants   *New quadrants*

upper right	upper left	permanent teeth		deciduous teeth	
lower right	lower left	quadrant 1	quadrant 2	quadrant 5	quadrant 6
		quadrant 4	quadrant 3	quadrant 8	quadrant 7

The first digit represents the quadrant and the second the tooth number. So you end up with:

permanent teeth

18 17 16 15 14 13 12 11 | 21 22 23 24 25 26 27 28

48 47 46 45 44 43 42 41 | 31 32 33 34 35 36 37 38

deciduous teeth

55 54 53 52 51 | 61 62 63 64 65

85 84 83 82 81 | 71 72 73 74 75

So the tooth written as, for example, '18' is pronounced 'one eight'. The deciduous teeth are numbered 1 to 5 (equivalent to A to E). When reading off the teeth you start in the top left quadrant and proceed in a clockwise direction around the quadrants.

Examples of dental summaries

It will be seen that the patient in the second letter has mixed dentition, permanent as well as some deciduous teeth.

Example 18.1   Orthodontic summary – letter form

Thank you for referring this patient who presented with a mild Class II division I malocclusion with some crowding of both arches. I note that he has a class I buccal segment relationship on either side, the over-bite (OB) is increased and just incomplete, and the over-jet (OJ) is 5 mm. I am a little concerned about his oral hygiene and associated gingival condition and I would very much hope to keep treatment simple. In view of this and the fact that he does not have a genuinely severe malocclusion, I would be most grateful if you could undertake his treatment locally using removable applicances. As a first step, I would be grateful if you could investigate $\underline{|6}$ which may have recurrent caries. Providing this tooth is in good order I would be grateful if, following some oral hygiene instruction, you could extract all four first premolars $\frac{4|4}{4|4}$ and fit an upper removable appliance designed to retract the upper canines. I would be grateful if you could then treat him with removable appliances as follows:

1. A URA (upper removable appliance) to retract $3|3$ following the premolar extractions. An anterior bite plane should be used to reduce the over-bite during this phase of treatment.
2. A second appliance designed to reduce the over-jet. The acrylic should be trimmed anteriorly on appliance 1 to allow the upper incisors to unravel a little. Following over-jet reduction, a six-month period of retention is required.

Example 18.2   Orthodontic summary – letter form

Thank you for asking me to see this boy who presented with Class 1 malocclusion in the later mixed dentition with crowding in both arches and inadequate room for his canines. I note that he has unilateral cross-bite on the left side with slight displacement.

I would be grateful if you could fit an upper removable appliance incorporating an offset screw to move $|E$ buccally (turned once a week) in order to correct the cross-bite, and hence the displacement. I would suggest cribs on $6E|6E$ and a thin posterior bite plane and labial bow on $1|1$ only. I think the treatment will take about 9 months or so to complete. Upon fitting the appliance, could you extract the upper right and both lower first premolars as well as the upper left first deciduous molar $\frac{4|D}{4|4}$ and $|4$ as soon as it erupts.

Once the cross-bite has been corrected, I think the appliance should be left in place a little longer then, to await eruption of the upper canines, and if necessary these can be guided in.

Example 18.3 Oral surgery summary

Report on operation on mandible (injury involving fractures)

Upper and lower metal arch bars were wired directly to the teeth. This involved a metal bar being fixed directly to the teeth by a series of wire loops which were twisted around the teeth and the bar. A transnasal wire was passed. The procedure entailed the passing of a stainless steel wire from the splint across the floor of the nose doubled back on itself to the splint. The upper and lower arch bars were then wired directly to each other, thus immobilizing both upper and lower jaws in their correct position of dental occlusion.

An extra-oral approach was made through the laceration to the comminuted fractured mandible. Wound toilet and debridement was carried out. This involved removing of all extraneous matter, road dirt, glass particles and small spicules of non-vital bone.

The comminuted fractured fragments of the mandible were directly wired together to restore the continuity of the lower border of the mandible.

A coronoidectomy was performed. This involved the stripping of the temporalis muscle off the coronoid process of the mandible and utilizing it as a bone graft to reinforce the fracture site. With the mandible reconstructed and immobilized, the remainder of the operation was performed by our plastic surgery colleagues who will provide a detailed report.

Example 18.4 Oral surgery summary

Later report on the patient in Example 18.3 after her attendance at Outpatients.

The patient was seen in the clinic this morning. She complained that she was unable to occlude her teeth together properly and thus was unable to bite crusty rolls, apples etc because her teeth did not meet in the original position. Her original dentures did not fit since the operation and her eating problems were compounded by the fact that due to loss of sensation to her lips she was continually biting her cheek, and food once in her mouth, continually spilled out.

On examination there was a very obvious left-sided facial asymmetry mainly due to an infrazygomatic depression resulting from loss of soft-tissue to that side of the face. Her mandibular opening was still somewhat reduced. The intercisal distance was measured at 3 cm. On opening there was marked deviation of the jaw to the left-hand side which in the main prevented the patient from achieving a centric occlusion (a position of maximum intercuspal interdigitation of the teeth).

The cosmetic state of her dentition is poor and requires extensive conservation and construction of new partial upper and lower dentures. There is a large area of decreased sensation to the lower lip extending back along the jaw line on the left, although there is some recovery of function to the lower lip. The upper lip and side of nose continue to be palsied.

Example 18.5   Left parotid sialogram

> The examination is abnormal. There is paucity of ducts in the superior portion of the parotid gland and those ducts which do show filling are displaced and show some scalloping. The appearances are suggestive of a mass lesion in the upper portion of the parotid gland. The most likely diagnosis would be some form of parotid tumour. The remaining ducts in the lower portion of the gland show no abnormalities.

Dental prostheses and appliances

bows (labial, face)
bridges
clasps (ball ended)
cribs (Adam's)
crowns
dentures (cobaltchrome overlay)
glass ionomer wear
implants (Brännermark)
splints (acrylic – may be heat cured, metal cap, gunning)
wires – circumferential, interdental eyelet, transosseous

Dental formulations

Mouthwashes, calcium supplements, sodium fluoride and local anaesthetics are used widely in dentistry and you can look these up in the *British National Formulary*.

A sialogram

A sialogram is an X-ray examination of the salivary ducts performed by injecting a radiopaque contrast (often referred to as a dye) into the duct. The parotid glands are the largest of the three main pairs of salivary glands. The parotid duct, sometimes called Stensen's duct, runs forward in the cheek and opens on the inside surface of the cheek opposite the second molar of the upper jaw.

Glossary of terms used in dentistry and oral surgery

Term	Meaning
amalgam	alloy of mercury with another metal which may be used in dental fillings.
apicectomy	excision of the apical portion of a tooth root through an incision into the overlying alveolar bone.

Term	*Meaning*
articulator	a device that simulates movement of the temperomandibular joint or mandible. Study models may be put on a semiadjustable articulator.
attrition	friction, wearing out.
axio- (word element)	in dentistry used in reference to the long axis of a tooth.
bicuspid	premolar tooth.
bruxism	gnashing, grinding or clenching of teeth usually during sleep. May be due to dental problems or emotional stress.
buccal	directed towards the cheek.
caries	decay in teeth.
cementoma	mass of cementum lying free at apex of tooth, probably a reaction to injury.
coronoid	in oral surgery refers to the coronoid process of the mandible.
cusp	pointed or rounded projection such as the crown of a tooth.
diastema	space between two adjacent teeth in the same dental arch.
distobuccal	pertaining to the distal and buccal surfaces of a tooth.
edentulous	without teeth.
endontics	branch of dentistry concerned with cause (aetiology), prevention, diagnosis and treatment of conditions that affect the tooth pulp, root and periapical tissues.
equilibration	achievement of balance between opposing elements.
frenulum or frenum	a restraining structure, commonly refers to the frenum of the tongue which, if it is too short, causes tongue tie. In dentistry may also refer to the frenum of the lip, a fold of mucous membrane connecting the inside of each lip to the corresponding gum.
furcation	forking.
genial	pertaining to the chin.
glossal	pertaining to the tongue.
gnathic	pertaining to the jaw.
interdigitation	interlocking parts by finger-like process.
labial	pertaining to the lip.

Term	Meaning
lingually	towards the tongue.
mental	pertaining to the chin.
mesiodens	small supernumerary tooth usually in the palate (pl. mesiodentes).
occlusal	pertaining to closure, applied usually to the masticating surfaces of the premolar and molar teeth.
orthodontics	branch of dentistry concerned with the prevention and correction of the malocclusion of teeth.
orthognathics	science dealing with the cause and treatment of malposition of the bones of the jaw.
overbite	vertical overlap between upper and lower incisor teeth when jaws are closed normally.
overjet	horizontal overlap between upper and lower teeth when jaws are closed normally.
periodontist	one who specializes in the treatment and surgery of the periodontium.
plaque	deposit of material on surface of tooth; can lead to periodontal disease.
pogonion	the anterior mid point of the chin.
prognathism	abnormal protrusion of the jaw.
pterygoid process	either of the two processes of the sphenoid bone.
retrognathia	under development of the maxilla and/or mandible.
stomatitis	inflammation of the mucosa of the mouth.
sulcus	gingival sulcus, space between tooth and gum.
trismus	spasm of the masticatory muscles with difficulty in opening the mouth.
zygomatic process	a projection from the frontal or temporal bone or maxilla by which they articulate with the cheek bone.

Some oral surgery operations

Oral surgery operations can be done under a local or general anaesthetic but would probably be done under a general anaesthetic if part of a list in the main theatres.

Exploration operations are normally carried out in cases of infection, tumour or other abnormalities.

Name	*Procedure*
alveolectomy	excision of the alveolar process to aid the removal of teeth and in preparation of the mouth for dentures.
apicectomy	excision of the apical portion of a tooth root through an incision into the overlying alveolar bone.
clearance	removal of all remaining teeth.
coronoidectomy	removal of the coronoid process of the mandible.
drainage masseteric abscess	abscess pertaining to the masseter muscle, the muscle that closes the jaw.
exploration of temperomandibular joint	temperomandibular joint (TMJ) is between the mandible and temporal bone. There may be dysfunction of the TMJ marked by pain, clicking, grinding and stiffness.
exploration of submental region	submental = under chin area.
frenectomy	excision of the frenum.
genioplasty and reduction right angle of jaw	genioplasty is a plastic surgery operation to chin.
gingivectomy	excision of all loose infected and diseased gum tissue to eradicate periodontal infection.
intermaxillary fixation of mandible, reduction and wiring mandible	performed in cases of fractured jaw.
osteotomy	surgical cutting of a bone. Types done in oral surgery are: Le Fort osteotomy bimaxillary forward sliding sagittal split Schuchardt Wassmund.
removal dental cyst	cyst usually of developmental origin associated with an unerupted tooth.
removal of impacted 'eights'	removal of impacted wisdom teeth, all four $\dfrac{8\mid 8}{8\mid 8}$
removal of bony exostosis	removal of a benign bony growth.
removal of mesiodens	mesiodens is a small supernumerary tooth usually in the palate.
sulcoplasty with skin grafting	plastic surgery operation on lining of mouth.

Chapter 19
Plastic Surgery and Burns

This chapter contains samples of plastic surgery letters and a report on a patient in a Burns Unit. Common names of skin grafts are given as well as some muscles, tendons and nerves in the hand and wrist. Finally there are examples of some plastic surgery operations.

Plastic surgery is the replacement, alteration or restoration of visible parts of the body, and may be performed for structural or cosmetic purposes. Skin grafting is the most common procedure in plastic surgery.

Plastic surgery summaries with explanations of terms used

The following examples are all in letter form. An indication of the area of body in question is given.

Example 19.1   Nose

This patient had a recurrent basal cell carcinoma (BCC) excised from his nose under local anaesthetic. The frozen section showed an early squamous cell carcinoma with a complete clearance. The deficit was covered with a **bilobed flap**. When seen in the clinic the flap looked fine and we have made arrangements to review him in six months.

Example 19.2   Pelvis

This patient was admitted with a left ischial pressure sore. He has been paraplegic since childhood. The pressure sore was infected and frequent dressings were required before operation was performed. A **rotation flap** was used from his left buttock. The donor defect had a skin graft which took some time to heal but when this was satisfactory he was discharged home.

Example 19.3   Nose and ear

This patient had an excision of **keratosis** from the right **nasolabial fold** and a sebaceous cyst from the **pre-auricular region**. He had previously had a benign cyst excised from the **glabellar** area.

Example 19.4   Nose

> This patient underwent correction of her nose tip + **ala**. She has a grossly
> deformed tip and alar cartilage which were corrected by an open technique.
> She is expected to have a satisfactory appearance following this procedure.

Example 19.5   Eyebrow and calf

> This patient had a cellular naevus removed from the right eyebrow and
> multiple **dermatofibromata** from the left calf. We will let you know the
> histology when it is to hand.

Example 19.6   Eyelid and upper lip

> This patient had a **seborrhoeic** keratosis excised from her left inner **canthus**
> and a basal cell carcinoma from her upper lip. Unfortunately histology
> showed the basal cell carcinoma had extended to the lateral excision
> margin so we will have to do a further excision to clear this.

Example 19.7   Skin

> This lady was admitted with a massive haematoma on her right shin
> following an injury. The haematoma was evacuated and the **necrotic skin**
> was excised under a general anaesthetic. The defect was covered with a
> **split skin graft**. She made an excellent recovery and was allowed home
> when the graft had fully taken.

Explanation of terms used in Examples 19.1–19.7

ala   (vomer alar) winglike structure of bone forming septum of the nose.

bilobed flap   (Zimany's bilobed flap) surgical flap with large lobe to fill
  primary defect with smaller lobe to fill secondary defect produced by
  mobilization of the large lobe.

canthus   the angle at either end of the fissure between the eyelids.

dermatofibromata   fibrous tumour-like nodule of the dermis.

glabella   area between the eyebrows.

keratosis   horny growth such as wart.

nasolabial fold   fold between nose and lip.

necrotic skin   dead skin.

pre-auricular region   area in front of auricle of the ear.

rotation flap   pedicle flap (full-thickness skin attached by pedicle) whose
  width is increased by transforming the distal edge into a curved line.

seborrhoeic   common form of keratosis.

split skin graft   skin graft consisting of only the superficial layer of the skin.

Plastic surgery summaries – the hand and wrist with explanations of terms used

Example 19.8   Finger/thumb

This little boy was in hospital about six weeks ago when he underwent **pollicization** of his left index finger, that is, it was moved into position where his left thumb would normally be, to act as a thumb.

The operation was uneventful and he has healed up nicely. His splints have been removed and at this stage his finger is quite stable. Unfortunately no flexor tendons are present in this left index finger and therefore he will not be able to flex the finger. In time he will need a flexor tendon graft to get movement in the finger.

Example 19.9   Finger

This patient was admitted for **fasciectomy** for **Dupuytren's contracture** of his left little finger. He had a reasonably good correction of his PIP joint. We shall keep an eye on his progress.

Example 19.10   Wrist

This patient was admitted as an emergency with a laceration to his left wrist which he accidentally cut on broken porcelain. His wound was explored under general anaesthetic and his **flexor carpi radialis** tendon was found to be completely divided. He was lucky to save his median nerve. The tendon was repaired and he made an uneventful recovery.

Example 19.11   Finger

This boy was re-admitted and **tenolysis** to his right little finger was undertaken. The tendons were completely stuck down to the soft tissues. The tendons were excised and a **Silastic** spacer was inserted extending from the distal phalanx to the palm.

He was also short of skin which was covered by a transposition flap raised from the dorsal aspect of the finger and the defect on the dorsum of the little finger was covered with a split skin graft. We shall keep a very close eye on him to mobilize his finger and will re-admit him for tendon grafting in the very near future.

Explanation of terms used in Examples 19.8–19.11

Dupuytren's contracture shortening, thickening and fibrosis of the palmar fascia producing a flexion deformity of the finger.

fasciectomy excision of a sheet or band of fibrous tissue (fascia) lying deep to the skin.

flexor carpi radialis tendon in wrist.

pollicization surgical construction of a thumb.

Silastic trademark for polymeric silicone substance in surgical prostheses.

tenolysis release of stuck tendons.

Anatomical names in fingers, hands and wrist

Many plastic surgery operations are carried out on the hand following injury, or for the correction of congenital abnormalities. It is useful to be familiar with the names of the muscles, tendons and nerves in the fingers, hand and wrist.

Fingers
dorsal and palmar interossei
extensor digitorum communis
extensor indicis propius.
flexor digitorum profundus (FDP)
flexor digitorum sublimis (FDS)
lumbricals   small muscles deeply placed in the palm of the hand
volar interossei = palmar interossi.

Thumb
abductor pollicis longus
abductor pollicis brevis
adductor pollicis
extensor pollicis brevis
extensor pollicis longus
flexor pollicis brevis (FPB)
flexor pollicus longus (FPL)
opponens pollicis
thenar eminence   three small muscles forming the fleshy part of the ball of the thumb.

Wrist
abductor pollicis longus
extensor carpi radialis brevis
extensor carpi radialis longus
extensor carpi ulnaris (ECU)
flexor carpi radialis
flexor carpi ulnaris.

Nerves
cutaneous nerve
interosseous nerve
median nerve
radial nerve
ulnar nerve.

Other useful terms used in plastic surgery

adipectomy   another name for a lipectomy.

cicatrix   a scar, new tissue formed in the healing of a wound.

columella nasi   a fleshy distal margin of the nasal septum.

commissura labiorum oris   commissure of lips of mouth – i.e. junction of the upper and lower lips at either side of the mouth.

keloid   sharply irregularly shaped progressively enlarging scar due to formation of excessive amount of collagen in the corium (dermis) during the healing process.

lipectomy   excision of mass of subcutaneous fatty (adipose). Sometimes called adipectomy.

plication   taking in of tucks in any structure.

syndactly   a common congenital anomaly of hand (or foot) with persistence of webbing between the digits.

Plastic surgery operations

The following lists some procedure/operations, not listed elsewhere, that may be applied to plastic surgery.

Abdominal

The following procedures are very much the same but expressed in different terms:

abdominal lipectomy
apronectomy
gastric plication
reduction abdominoplasty

Breast

mastopexy
reduction mammoplasty
silicone implants

Hand

flexor tenolysis of finger
index pollicization

Ear

correction of bat ears
otoplasty
pinnaplasty

Nose

rhinophyma repair
rhinoplasty
septoplasty or septorhinoplasty

Other operations

Name	Procedure
blepharoplasty	plastic surgery of the eyelids.
cheiroplasty	plastic surgery on the hand.
dermabrasion	surgical removal of epidermis and dermis by mechanical means such as sandpaper, wire brushes etc. Used to remove scars, tattoos, pigmented naevi and fine wrinkles.
meloplasty	plastic surgery of the cheek.
Z-plasty	operative release of contractures in which a Z-shaped incision is made.

Skin grafts

A skin graft is a piece of skin which is implanted in places where skin has been lost through burn injury or surgical excision. For permanent grafts, skin is taken from the patient's own body (or identical twin) to prevent tissue rejection. For temporary cover, skin from another person (or an animal) may be used for large burn areas to prevent serious fluid loss. Some common skin grafts are:

allograft
autograft (autologous graft)
bilobed graft
fascicular graft
Fromberg graft
meshed graft
pedicled graft
pinch graft
split skin graft (SSG)
sponge graft
stent graft
Thiersch graft
tube graft
Wolfe graft

Burns

Many patients suffering from severe burns have smoke inhalation injuries as well. Severe cases are nursed on a ventilator and are under the care of the anaesthetist as well as the plastic surgeon. Blood gases have to be carefully monitored, intravenous infusions maintained and urine output assessed. There is a great risk of shock, dehydration and septicaemia.

Pressure garments are used in many cases of burns, frequently Jobst garments.

Classification of burns and the rule of nines

Burns may be classified according to the depth of tissue damage and/or according to the extent of body surface damaged. Thus:

first degree burns are partial-thickness burns, involving only the surface epidermis;
second degree burns involve the epidermis and some of the dermis;
third degree burns are full thickness burns and involves all skin layers, being the most severe grade.

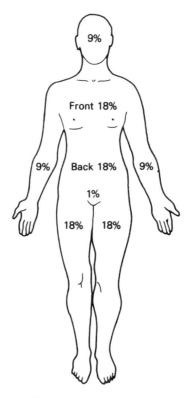

Fig. 19.1   Rule of nines. (*Source* Willatts 1987.)

There is also a rule known as the 'rule of nines' which is a formula for quickly estimating the extent of body surface affected by burns. This is best explained by Fig. 19.1.

Example of burns summary with explanation of terms used

Example 19.12 Burns summary – letter form

> This lady was transferred as an emergency following a road traffic accident in which she sustained extensive deep burns to 25% of the body surface involving mainly the right side.
>
> She was found to have full-thickness burns to the right hand, right forearm, right upper arm, right side of the face, right side of the neck, whole of right leg, patches on the left knee and left hand and forearm. The circulation to the right forearm was impaired and emergency **escharotomies** were performed to release the tourniquet-like effect. Large amounts of plasma volume expander and blood were given and she was prepared for surgery.
>
> An attempt was made to excise all the burned areas down to healthy tissue and resurface them with skin grafts taken from unburned areas. Good progress was made initially but unfortunately the wounds became heavily infected and there was much loss of skin graft and, in fact on two occasions serious septicaemia occurred. Fortunately, the septic episodes responded to high-dose antibiotics but it proved difficult to maintain adequate nutrition and morale.
>
> Some surgical procedures undertaken: Excision of all burns down to deep dermis and fat meshed skin grafts taken from left thigh, left lower leg and abdomen, applied to raw areas.
>
> Change of dressings, wounds clean, although finger tips necrotic, not viable to the level of proximal interphalangeal joints.
>
> **ectropion** of the right eye corrected with insertion of a **Wolfe graft** into the lower lid.

Explanation of terms used in Example 19.12

    ectropion   an everted eyelid.
    eschar   is a slough produced by a thermal burn; **escharotomies** cutting into the slough, frequently performed on burns patients.
    Wolfe graft   full thickness graft, frequently taken from behind the ear.

Appendices

Bibliography

Sources of figures

Gibson J. (1981) *Modern Physiology and Anatomy for Nurses*. 2 ed. Blackwell Scientific Publications, Oxford.

Leatham A., Bull C. and Braimbridge M.V. (1991) *Lecture Notes on Cardiology*. 3 ed. Blackwell Scientific Publications, Oxford.

Levison H. (1991) *Textbook for Dental Nurses*. 7 ed. Blackwell Scientific Publications, Oxford.

Moffat D.B. and Mottram R.F. (1987) *Anatomy and Physiology for Physiotherapists*. 2 ed. Blackwell Scientific Publications, Oxford.

Willatts S.M. (1987) *Lecture Notes on Fluid and Electrolyte Balance*. 2 ed. Blackwell Scientific Publications, Oxford.

Useful sources of reference

British National Formulary (BNF)
Published twice-yearly jointly by the British Medical Association and the Royal Pharmaceutical Society of Great Britain.

The Hospital and Health Services Year Book and Directory of Hospital Suppliers
Published annually by The Institute of Health Services Management.

The Medical Directory
Published annually by Longman Group UK Ltd. A directory of all the qualified medical doctors in the UK plus names and addresses for Regional Health Authorities, hospitals, Royal Colleges, medical societies and institutions and other useful bodies.

Monthly Index of Medical Specialities (MIMS)
A monthly magazine listing of all proprietary drugs and formulations with details of new compounds.

A good medical dictionary is also of use.

Useful Addresses

Association of Health Centre and Practice
    Adminstrators
14 Princes Gate
London SW7 1PU

Association of Medical Secretaries, Practice
    Administrators and Receptionists Ltd
    (AMSPAR)
Tavistock House North
Tavistock Square
London WC1H 9LN

British Medical Association (BMA)
BMA House
Tavistock Square
London WC1H 9JP

British United Provident Association
    (BUPA)
24/27 Essex Street
London WC2R 3AX

Committee on Safety of Medicines
Market Towers
1 Nine Elms Lane
London SW8 5NQ

Department of Health
Richmond House
79 Whitehall
London SW1A 2NS

Department of Social Security
Richmond House
79 Whitehall
London SW1A 2NS

General Medical Council (GMC)
44 Hallam Street
London W1N 6AE

Health Education Authority
Hamilton House
Mabledon Place
London WC1H 9TX

Health Services Superannuation Division
Hesketh House

200–220 Broadway
Fleetwood
Lancs FL7 8LG

Hospital Savings Association
30 Lancaster Gate
London W2 3LT

Institute of Health Services Management
75 Portland Place
London W1N 4AN

Medical Defence Union Ltd
3 Devonshire Place
London W1N 2AE

Medical Protection Society Ltd
50 Hallam Street
London W1N 6DE

Medical Research Council (MRC)
20 Park Crescent
London W1N 4AL

Nuffield Foundation
Nuffield Lodge
Regent's Park
London NW1 4RS

Royal College of General Practitioners
    (RCGP)
14 Prince's Gate
Hyde Park
London SW7 1PU

Royal College of Midwives (RCM)
15 Mansfield Street
London W1M 0BE

Royal College of Nursing (RCN)
20 Cavendish Square
London W1M 0AB

Royal College of Obstetricians and
    Gynaecologists (RCOG)
27 Sussex Place
Regent's Park
London NW1 4RG

Royal College of Physicians
11 St Andrew's Place
London NW1 4LE

Royal College of Surgeons of England
35 Lincoln's Inn Fields
London WC2A 3PN

Royal Society of Medicine (RSM)
1 Wimpole Street
London W1M 8AE

United Kingdom Central Council for
        Nursing, Midwifery and Health Visting
        (UKCC)
23 Portland Place
London W1N 3AF

World Health Organization (WHO)
Geneva
Switzerland

Alphabetical Word Elements and Terms

The main purpose of this chapter is to help you to look up terms in a medical dictionary with which you are not familiar – and may not have been heard distinctly when audiotyping. Therefore, words listed are those whose pronunciation and spelling are different or difficult, words which sound similar, and other words thought to be generally useful.

It is worthwhile to remember that some words have a silent first letter such as those beginning 'gn', 'ps', and 'pt', examples are gnathic, psoriasis and ptosis. Words starting 'ph' are pronounced as starting with 'f', e.g. phimosis, and those starting with 'pht' as 'th' e.g. phthisis; 'coel' is pronounced 'seel', e.g. coeliac. Some words beginning with a 'c' or 'k' sound the same, e.g. 'cal', 'kal', 'cat' and 'kat', and also those beginning with a 'c' or 's', e.g. 'cil' and 'sil'. An 'i' or a 'y' as the second letter in a word is difficult to distinguish, e.g. 'dis' and 'dys'; 'chon' and 'con' can also sound the same. A 'W' in some proper nouns may be pronounced as a 'v'; examples are Weber (test), Weil (disease), Wertheim (operation) and Werner (syndrome). It will be seen that this can make looking up an unfamiliar term more difficult. Whilst Chapter 6 gives prefixes and suffixes, which should be useful for the spelling and understanding of many terms, this appendix will provide an additional aid. Word elements and their meanings are given before listing the relevant terms.

It is usually possible when using a comprehensive medical dictionary to find, for example, a specific operation under 'Operation', or a specific syndrome under 'Syndrome' and this applies to many other general terms such as muscles, signs and reflexes etc. If an American dictionary is used it must be noted that in vowel combinations of 'ae' and 'oe' the letters 'a' and 'o' are omitted so that oedema becomes 'edema', oesophagus 'esophagus' and haemo becomes 'hemo'. There are other differences in spelling but not so significant as to hinder the finding of a word.

Latin is denoted by (L) and Greek by (Gk).

 A *Word elements*

a- without, not (an before a vowel) (L)
ab- from, off, away from (L)
abdomin(o)- abdomen (L)
acanth(o)- sharp, spine, thorn (Gk)
acromio- acromion (Gk)
actino- ray, radiation (Gk)
aero- air, gas (Gk)

amyl(o)- starch (Gk)
andr(o)- male, masculine (Gk)
anky(o)- bent, crooked (Gk)
antero- anterior, in front of (Gk)
asthen(o)- weak, weakness (Gk)
atel(o)- incomplete, imperfectly developed (Gk)

Some terms listed alphabetically

abdominoperineal
acanthoma
acetabulum
acetic acid
acetone
acetyl
acetylcholine
achalasia
achlorhydria
achromia
acidosis
acini
aclasia
acromegaly
actinic
adnexal
aerophagy
agranulocytosis
ala (n), alar (adj)
aldosteronism
alkalosis
allogenic
alphafetoprotein
Alzheimer's disease
amenorrhoea
amyloidosis
amytrophic
anaerobic
anaphylaxis
anencephalic

androgen
aneurysm
anisocytosis
ankylosing
anterolateral
Apgar score
aphagia
aphakia
aphasia
aphonia
apnoeic
apophyseal
aqueous
arachnoid
Aran-Duchenne
arrhythmia
arteriosclerosis
arytenoid
Aschoff's bodies
asphyxia
asthenia
atelectasis
atherosclerosis
atony
atopy (n), atopic (adj)
atresia
atrophy (n), atrophic (adj)
auricle
auscultation
azygos

B Word elements

bili- bile (L)
bio- life, living (Gk)
blasto- bud, budding (Gk)
brachi(o)- arm (L and Gk)
brachy- short (Gk)

Some terms listed alphabetically

bacteriuria
balanitis
Bartholin's cyst/duct/gland
basilic
basophils

Bence–Jones protein
Berger's paraesthesia
bicipital
bicornuate
Bier's block

bifascicular block
bifurcation
bilirubinaemia
Billroth's operation
biopsies
blastomycosis
blepharitis
BM Stix
Bouchard's nodes
bougie
brachial
brachycephalic
bradycardia

branchial
bronchiectasis
bruit
bruxism
buccal
buccinator muscle
Budd–Chiari syndrome
Buerger's disease
bulbar
bulla
bundle branch block
β-thalassaemia

C Word elements

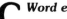

cervi(o)- neck, cervix (L)
cheil(o)- lip (Gk)
cheir(o)- hand (Gk)
chromat(o)- colour, chromatin (Gk)
coeli(o)- abdomen, through the abdominal wall (Gk)
cry(o)- cold (Gk)
cyt(o)- a cell (Gk)

Some terms listed alphabetically

cachexia
caecum (n), caecal (adj)
café au lait spot
calcaemia
calcaneus
calcareous
callus
calyces
cancellous
cancerous
canthus
caput succedaneum
carina
carotid
carpus
catecholamine
cauda equina
caudal
cavernous haemangioma
cellulitis
cerebrospinal
cervicovesical
Charcot's joint
Charcot Marie Tooth
cheiloplasty
cheirospasm
chiasma
choanal

cholelithiasis
cholesterol
chondroma
chordee
chorea
chorionic gonadotrophin
choroid plexus
chromatopsia
cicatrical tissue
ciliary
cirrhosis
clonus
coeliac disease
colectomy
colostomy
concha
coracoid
cord
coronoid
cor pulmonale
corpus
costophrenic
creatinine
cricoid
cri-du-chat syndrome
Crohn's disease
cryo-coagulation
cyanotic

cystocele (cystocoele)
cytopenia

cytotoxic

D Word elements

dacry(o)- tears or the lacrimal (lachrymal) apparatus of the eye (Gk)
dolich(o)- long (Gk)
dors(o)- the back, dorsal aspect (L)

Some terms listed alphabetically

dacryocystitis
debridement
decidua
dehiscence
demyelination
desquamation
de Quervain's
dialysis
diaphragmatic
diaphysis
diastasis
diathesis
Dipstix
diphtheria
diplopia
disseminated intravascular coagulation
diuresis/diuretic
diurnal
diverticulitis

dolichocephalic
dorsiflexion
Dubowitz assessment
ductus arteriosus
Dupuytren's contracture
dyscrasia
dysdiadochokinesia
dysergia
dyskaryotic
dyskinesia
dysmorphic
dysphagia
dysphasia
dysphonia
dysplasia
dyspnoeic
dystocia
dystonia
dystrophy

E Word elements

ect(o)- external, outside (Gk)
enter(o)- intestine (Gk)
ento- within, inner (Gk)
epi- upon (Gk)
erythro- red, erythrocyte (Gk)
eu- normal, good, well, easy (Gk)

Some terms listed alphabetically

ecchymoses
eclampsia
ectasia
ectocervix
ectopic, ectopia, ectopy
ectropion
eczema
edentulous
electrophoresis
emphysematous
empyema
endothelial
enterocolitis

entropion
enzyme
eosinophilia
epicanthic folds
epicardial fat pad
epididymo-orchitis
epiphyseal
epileptiform
episiotomy
epispadias
epistaxis
epithelial
erysipelas

erythematous
erythropoiesis
escharotomy
ethmoiditis
euthyroid
exacerbation

excitation
exophthalmos
exostosis
extrapyramidal
extravasation
exudate

F Word elements

faci(o)- face (L)
fibr(o)- fibre, fibrous (L)

Some terms listed alphabetically

fabella
facies
facioscapulohumeral
faecolith
Fallot's tetralogy
falx cerebri
fascia
fasciitis
fasciculation
fauces
fibrillation

fibromuscular
fissure
fistula
flaccid
flexor
flexure
flocculation
fontanelle
fremitus
frenulum
fructosamine

G Word elements

genito- relating to organs of reproduction (L)
ger-, gero-, geronto- old age, the aged, the elderly (Gk)
gingivo- gingival (pertaining to the gums) (L)

Some terms listed alphabetically

galactosaemia
gastrocnemius
gastroschisis
geneticist
genitourinary
geriatrician
Gilles de la Tourette syndrome
gingivoglossitis
ginglymus joints
glaucoma
glia
glioma
Glisson's capsule

glomerulonephritis
gluteal
glycaemia
glycosuria
gnathic
gonadotrophin
gouty tophus
gravida
grommet
Guillain-Barré syndrome
Guthrie test
gynaecomastia
gyrus

H Word elements

heli(o)- sun (Gk)
hemi- half (Gk)
heter(o)- other, dissimilar (Gk)
hidr(o)- sweat (Gk)
hol(o)- entire, whole (Gk)
homeo- similar, same, unchanging (Gk)
homo- same, similar (Gk)

Some terms listed alphabetically

Haelan tape
haemangioma
haematopoiesis
haemolytic
haemorrhoid
Harrison's sulcus (pl. sulci)
Hartmann's pouch
Hegar's dilators, sign
hemiparesis
hepatic
Herberden's nodes
herniorrhaphy
herpetic
hidroschesis
Hirschsprung's disease
hologynic
homeostatis
homogeneous
homogenous
homozygous

hyaline
hydatid of Morgagni
hydatidiform mole
hydramnios
hydrocephalic
17-hydroxycorticosteroids
hyoid
hyperaemia
hyperemesis gravidarum
hyperkalaemia
hyperkinetic
hypnotherapy
hypocalcaemia
hypochondrium
hyponatraemia
hypophysis
hypospadias
hypothenar eminence
hypoxia

I Word elements

idio- self, peculiar to a substance or organism (Gk)
ile(o)- ileum (L)
ili(o)- ilium (L)
infra- beneath (L)
ischi(o)- ischium (Gk)
iso- equal, alike, same (Gk)

Some terms listed alphabetically

ichthyosis
ictal
icterus
idiopathic
IgA deficiency
ileum
ileus
ilium (n), iliac (adj)
immunoglobulin
incus
infarction
infraspinous
inguinal
inspissated

intercondylar
interosseous
interphalangeal
interstitial
intertrochanteric
intima
introitus
intubation
intussusception
ischaemia
ischial (spine, tuberosity)
isotonic
isthmus

J Word element

juxta- situated near, adjoining (L)

Some terms listed alphabetically

Jadasshon (naevus of)
jejunostomy

Jobst garments
Joule

jugular juxtaposition
junctura

K Word elements

karyo- nucleus (Gk)
kerat(o)- horny tissue, cornea (Gk)
kine, kinesi(o)- movement (Gk)
koila- hollowed, concave (Gk)

Some terms listed alphabetically

Kahn's test
kalaemia
Kaposi's sarcoma
karyotype
keloid
keratinization
keratitis
kernicterus

ketosteroids
kinetic
Klinefelter's syndrome
koilonychia
Koplik's spots
kraurosis
kyphotic

L Word elements

laevo- left (L)
lal- speech, babbling (Gk)
laparo- loin or flank, abdomen (Gk)
lepto- slender, delicate (Gk)
lien(o)- spleen (L) (more commonly splen(o))
logo- words, speech (Gk)
lymph(o)- lymph, lymphoid tissue, lymphatics, lymphocytes (L)

Some terms listed alphabetically

lacunate ligament
laevorotation
lalopathology
lamella
lamina
Langerhans (islets of)
laparotomy
laryngeal
latissimus dorsi
leiomyoma
lentigo maligna
leptocephalus
leucocytosis or leukocytosis
leukoplakia

lichenification
lienculus
linea alba
lipids
liquor
lithiasis
lochia
logokophosus
lumbrical
lupus erythematosis
luxation
lymphocytosis
lysis

M Word elements

mega- large (Gk)
mening(o)- meninges, membrane (Gk)
mero- 1. part, 2. thigh (Gk)
meta- change, transformation, exchange, or after, next (Gk)
metra- metro- uterus (Gk)
mono- one, single, limited to one part (Gk)
myring(o)- tympanic membrane (L)

Some terms listed alphabetically

macerated
macrophages
macula
macules
malacia
malleolus
malleus
Mallory-Weiss tear/syndrome
masseter
mastitis
mastoiditis
matrix
megacolon
melaena
meniscus
menorrhagia
meralgia
mesenteric
mesothelioma
metaphysis
metaplasia
metastasis
methyl testosterone

metopic suture
metritis
microsomal antibodies
migraine
mittelschmerz
moiety
monoamine oxidase
morbilliform
Moro reflex
morphoeic
mosaicism
mucous (n)
mucus (adj)
myalgia
myasthenia gravis
myeloma
myelopathy
myoclonic
myofascial
myringotomy
myxoedema
myxoid

N Word elements

nano- dwarf, small size (Gk)
narco- stupor, stuporous state (Gk)
naso- nose (L)
necro- death (Gk)
neo- new, recent (Gk)
norm(o)- normal, usual conforming to the rule (L)
nyct(o)- night, darkness (Gk)

Some terms listed alphabetically

nabothian cysts/follicles
naevoxanthoendothelioma
naevus flammeus
nanogram
nanoid
narcolepsy
nasopharyngeal
nephrotic syndrome
neonates
neurofibromatosis

neutropenia
neutrophil
normotensive
nuchal
nucleus pulposus
nulliparous
nummular
nyctalopia
nystagmus

O Word elements

ob- against, in front of, toward (L)
ocul(o)- eye (L)
omphal(o)- umbilicus (Gk)
onco- tumour, swelling mass (Gk)
oneir(o)- dream (Gk)

onych(o)- the nails (Gk)
orth(o)- straight, normal, correct (Gk)
oscillo- oscillation (L)
ovari(o)- ovary (L) (also oophor(o) (Gk))

Some terms listed alphabetically

obturator
occipital
occipitoanterior
occiput
oculomotor
odontoid
oesophagus (n),
oesophageal (adj)
oligohydramnios
oligoptyalism
omentum
omphalocoele
oncology
oneirology
onychopathy

oophoritis
opisthotonos
orchitis
orthognathic
orthopnoea
os
os calcis
oscillopsia
osmosis
osteitis condensans ilii
osteophyte
otitis
ovariocyesis
oxyhaemoglobin
ozena

P *Word elements*

pachy- thick (Gk)
palat(o)- palate (L)
pali(n)- again, pathological repetition (Gk)
pancreato- pancreas (Gk)
para- beside, beyond, accessory to, apart from, against (Gk)
path(o)- disease (Gk)
pharyng(o)- pharynx (Gk)
phon(o)- sound, voice, speech (Gk)
phot(o)-light (Gk)
physio- nature, physiology, physical (Gk)
pilo- hair, composed of hair (L)
platy- broad, flat (Gk)
pleur(o)- pleura, rib, side (Gk)
pneumon- lung (Gk)
pod(o)- foot (Gk)
postero- the back, posterior to (L)
psosop(o)- face (Gk)
proto- first (Gk)
pseud(o)- false (Gk)
ptyal(o)- saliva (Gk)
pulmo- lung (L)
pyel(o)- renal pelvis (Gk)
pykn(o)- thick, compact, frequent (Gk)
pyle- portal vein (Gk)
pylor(o)- pylorus (Gk)
pyro- fire, heat (Gk)

Some terms listed alphabetically

pachydermia
palatoglossal

palindromic
pancreatogram

paraesthesia
paraplegia
parenchymal
parietal
paronychia
paroxysmal
parturition
pathogenic
pauciarticular
peau d'orange
perineal
peristalsis
peritoneal
peroneal muscle
petechial
petit mal
Pfannenstiel incision
phagocyte
phalanges
Phalen's sign
pharyngolaryngeal
phenylketonuria
phenylpyruvic acid
phimosis
phlebotomy
phlegm
phototherapy
phrenic
phthisis
physiotherapy
pia mater
pilonidal sinus
pineal
pinna
pisiform
plagiocephaly
plasma phoresis
platypelloid
platypodia
pleomorphic

pleuropericardial
pneumoperitoneum
poikilocytosis
pollicization
polycythaemia
polydactyly
polydipsia
porphyria
preputial
procidentia
proctitis
prognathic
prophylaxis
prosopospasm
prostatism
protocol
prurigo
psammoma
pseudocyesis
psittacosis
psoas muscle
psoriasis
psychosis
pterygium
pterygoid process
ptomaine
ptosis
ptyalin
pubarche
pudendal
puerperal
pulmonary
purpura
pyelonephritis
pylephlebitis
pyloric stenosis
pyosalpinx
pyrogen
pyuria

 R ## Word elements

rachi(o)- spine (Gk)
radio- ray, radiation, emission of radiant energy, radius (bone of forearm) (L)
rect(o)- rectum (L)
rheo- electric current, flow (as of fluids) (Gk)
rhizo- root (Gk)

Some terms listed alphabetically

rachitic
radiculogram
radiocarpal joint
radiopaque

radium
radius (n), radial (adj)
rales
Ramstedt' operation

Raynaud's disease
rectovaginal
rectus abdominis (muscle)
regimen
resuscitation
reticular
retinal
retrocaecal

rheostat
rhinophyma
rhizoid
rhonchus
Riedel's lobe/struma
Rose–Waaler test
rotator cuff
ruga, rugae

S Word elements

sangui- blood (L)
sapr(o)- rotten, putrid, decay, decayed material (Gk)
sarc(o)- flesh (Gk)
schist(o)- cleft, split (Gk)
schiz(o)- divided, division (Gk)
scirrho- hard (Gk)
scoli(o)- crooked, twisted (Gk)
scoto- darkness (Gk)
sial(o)- saliva, salivary gland (Gk)
sidero- iron (Gk)
sinistr(o)- left, left side (L)
spermato- seed, specifically used to refer to male germinal element (Gk)
spheno- wedge shaped, sphenoid bone (Gk)
sphygmo- the pulse (Gk)
splanchn(o)- viscus (viscera), splanchnic nerve (Gk)
spondy(o)- vertebra, vertebral column (Gk)
steat(o)- fat, oil (Gk)
sterco- faeces (L)
stern(o)- sternum (L & Gk)
steth(o)- chest (Gk)
supra- above (L)
syn- union, associated (Gk)

Some terms listed alphabetically

sacrococcygeal
sagittal
salicylates
salpinx
sanguineous
saphenous
saprophyte
sarcoidosis
scaphoid
schistocyte
schizophrenia
sciatic
scirrhous
scleroderma
scoliosis
scotoma
sebaceous
seborrhoeic
sella turcica

sequestrum
serology
sesamoid
Shirodkar suture
sialectasia
siccus
sideroblastic
sigmoid
silicosis
sinistrocardia
sinus arrhythmia
smegma
somatic
sphenoid
spherocytosis
sphincter
sphygmomanometer
Spitz–Holter valve
splanchnic

splenic
spondylosis
staphylococcal
steatorrhoea
Stein–Leventhal's syndrome
stercoral
sternomastoid
stethoscope
stoma
stroma

suprapubic
sycosis
symphysis
synarthrosis
syncytial knots
syndactyly
synechia
synergists
synkinesia
synovial

T Word elements

tachy- rapid, swift (Gk)
tars(o)- edge of eyelid, tarsus of foot, instep (Gk)
teno- tendon (Gk)
tetra- four (Gk)
therm(o)- heat (Gk)
thyro- thyroid (Gk)
tomo- a section, cutting (Gk)
trachel(o)- neck, necklike structure especially the uterine cervix (Gk)
tracheo- trachea (Gk)
trans- through, across, beyond (L)
troph(o)- food, nourishment (Gk)
typhl(o)- caecum, blindness (Gk)

Some terms listed alphabetically

tachypnoeic
tamponade
tardive
tarsorrhaphy
telangiectasis
tenesmus
tenosynovitis
tetanus
tetany
tetralogy
thalamus
thalassaemia
thallium
theca (n), thecal (adj)
thenar
therapeutic
thermocautery
thiamine
thrombocytopenic
thyrotoxicosis
tic douloureux
tinea
Tinel's sign
tinnitus
tomogram

tophaceous
trabeculated
trachelorrhaphy
tracheostomy
trachoma
transaminase
transurethral
trephine
trichomonas
trichosis
trifurcation
trigeminal
trigone
trimester
trismus
trisomy
trochanter
trochlear
trophic
tunica vaginalis
typmpanic
tympanites
typhlolexia
typhlolithiasis

U *Word elements*

ultra- beyond, excess (L)
uni- one (L)
ureter(o)- ureter (Gk)
urethr(o)- urethra (Gk)
uro- urine, urinary tract, urination (Gk)
uter(o)- uterus (L)

Some terms listed alphabetically

ultrasound
uniovular
uraemia
urea
ureteric
ureterocoele
urethritis
urethrocoele
urinalysis
urogram
uterosacral

V *Word elements*

vas(o)- vessel, duct (L)
ven, vene, veno- vein (L)
ventr(i) ventr(o)- belly, front, (anterior) aspect of the body, ventral aspect (L)
vertebr(o)- vertebra, spine (L)

Some terms listed alphabetically

vagal
valgus
vallecula
Valsalva's manoeuvre
varices
varicocoele
varicula
vas deferens
vasectomy
vasoocclusive
venepuncture
Ventouse extraction
ventral

ventricle
vertebrocostal
vertigo
vesical
villus (n), villous (adj)
virgo intacta
visceral
visceroptosis
vitiligo
volar interossei
Volkmann's contracture
volvulus
vomer

W *Some terms listed alphabetically*

Wegener's granulomatosis
Weil's disease
Werner's syndrome
Wertheim's operation
wheal

whorl
Wilm's tumour
Wolff–Parkinson–White syndrome
wryneck

X *Word elements*

xanth(o)- yellow (Gk)
xer(o)- dry, dryness (Gk)
xiph(o)- xiphoid process (Gk)

Some terms listed alphabetically

xanthelasma
xanthoma
xerosis

xiphocostal
Xylocaine

Z *Word elements*

zyg(o)- yoked, joined, a junction (Gk)
zym(o) enzyme, fermentation (Gk)

Some terms listed alphabetically

zygoma
zygote

zymotic
Z-plasty

Index